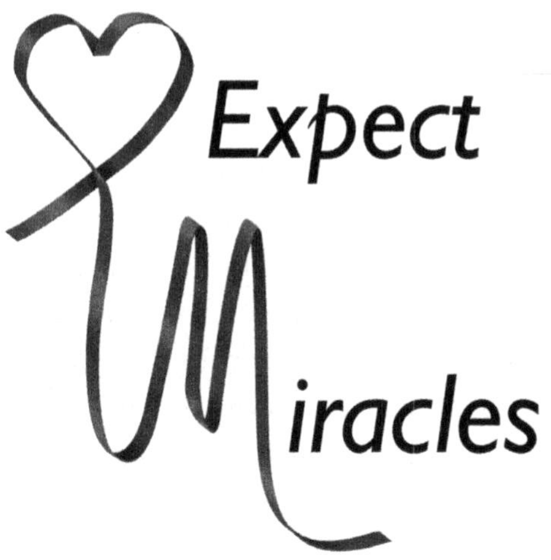

10 beautiful souls share stories of
Hope, Inspiration, and Transformation

Sue Dumais
in collaboration with
Kimberly Shuttleworth • Kelly Van Unen • Kent Smith
Diana Calvo • Rachel Shoniker • Delle Vaughan
Lisa Windsor • Kirsty Peckham • Joanne Sissons

Published by Heart Led Living Publishing Oct, 2017
ISBN: 9780995813021

Editor: Nina Shoroplova
Typeset: Greg Salisbury
Cover Design: Judith Mazari
Cover Graphic Art: Sarah Scheifele
Sue Dumais's Portrait Photographer: Adrienne Thiessen of Gemini Visuals Creative Photography

This book is a gift for the hearts of all humanity.

This book is a gift for the hearts of all humanity.

Testimonials

"Sue Dumais will challenge you to stand in your power, get out of your comfort zone and stand up for what you believe in. Sue's message comes from her heart. It will stop you from running and make you face the truth of who you are, and that will set you free."

Les Brown, World renowned Motivational Speaker, Best selling Author

"Sue Dumais and her Heart Led Living Community have had a huge influence on my life. Instead of being overwhelmed by doubt, I have learned to embrace the unknown with curiosity one step, one moment, one breath at a time. The stories within this collaborative book are a beautiful embodiment of all that being guided by your heart has to offer. Expect miracles!"

Marilyn R, Wilson, Freelance Writer, Published Author, Speaker

"One thing I found absolutely incredible about Sue is her intuition and powerful ability to have that resonate for my deepest growth. Sue is particularly amazing at reminding me what is soul inspired and what is not, and creating the space to be spirit led. I would highly recommend Sue to anyone looking to be more heart led in all that they are and do in the world."

Lara Kozan, Co-Founder YYoga & Nectar Juicery, Entrepreneur, Coach

"Mastery is what comes to mind when I think about Sue Dumais as a coach and intuitive healer. Through her masterful art I have become more confident in trusting, listening and being guided by my intuition, this has provided me with substantial growth personally and professionally."

Kate Muker, Conscious Diva, Entrepreneur, Speaker

Acknowledgements

We are deeply grateful for all the love and support of our families, friends and mighty companions walking beside us through the process of bringing this book to life.

Thank you to our publisher and writing coach, Julie Salisbury for guiding all of us into our hearts to bring our stories onto the pages of this book.

A big thank you to our editor and gentle shepherd, Nina Shoroplova for working with each of us individually to fine tune our stories and her ability to guide us to bring our vision together.

We are grateful for our loving, nurturing and sacred Heart Led Living community for providing a safe place for authentic expression, soulful conversations, deep healing and transformation. May we continue to grow together and unite our hearts in love for each other and our planet.

Contents

What to Expect? Miracles, of Course!

This book is a joining together of ten beautiful souls bravely sharing stories from their lives to inspire and empower others to be willing to face their fears, to feel and honour their feelings, to overcome adversity, and find meaning through their life's challenges. This book is infused with hope, inspiration, and insights that help all of us move through the darkness into the light. This book is a gift for humanity.

Albert Einstein said, "Live life as if everything is a miracle." The truth is *everything is a miracle* including you. We are meant to be celebrated.

Since 2012, Heart Led Living has become a global community of compassionate hearts, healers, intuitive coaches, lightworkers, and like-hearted individuals who are dedicated to follow their intuition and fulfil their heart's path. Three years ago, I began personally mentoring and training intuitive coaches, healers and lightworkers to embrace and enhance their innate gifts. We empower each other as we empower ourselves.

I hold a sacred container for our Heart Led Living community and in every moment I am willing to play my part. When I received the insight to write a collaborative book on *Expect Miracles* I was excited to co-create within our community. When I put out the call to my members and intuitive coaches and healers to author a book filled with stories of hope, inspiration, and miracles there was an overwhelming YES from these nine authors. They had a deep knowing they had a part to play in this project. They all stood up and said YES to their heart's call to participate.

This is a book of miracles. Miracles happen all the time. Many of us overlook, minimize, or underestimate the power of acknowledging and celebrating the miracles that occur in our lives. We don't want to toot our own horn or feel we are bragging. The truth is miracles are a natural side effect of being in alignment with our true authentic self and each one is meant to be celebrated.

The Birth of Heart Led Living

I have always been a seeker of truth and understanding. I always felt something deep inside calling me toward something bigger, something more. For the first half of my life I was terrified of the power held within me, yet that inner light always kept me going even in my darkest times.

I experienced some intense struggles with anorexia, bulimia, alcohol and substance abuse, unworthiness, self-sabotage, and a lot of pain and suffering. It all stemmed from my inner world and the chaotic storm of fear and anxiety in my head.

One day I happened upon the book *The Celestine Prophecy.* It was my first experience and memory that consciously created an opening in my mind and a realization that there was more to this thing called life. The door had been opened and the light of awareness came in, my limited thinking mind was challenged in a way that I couldn't go back to living in the darkness. I saw the light and I felt the call so deeply that I woke up and I was driven to find the meaning and purpose for my life.

Over the years I spent thousands and thousands of dollars and countless hours on self-help, personal growth, and spiritual development. I would attend a workshop and feel inspired and motivated to make changes, but within a few short days all that energy would dissolve. While I made many changes, received lots of aha moments and each one contributed in one way or another to my healing and awakening, there was still something missing. I was still seeking something I just wasn't finding. I wanted to make specific changes but I found my efforts too slow, and some of the changes were only temporary.

Even with the hundreds of books and workshops, I still struggled. I would experience these ebbs and flows, highs and lows, and eventually my energy would start to fade. That is when my ego mind would take over with thoughts of fear, doubt, procrastination, and self-sabotage. I was taking two steps forward and one step back. It was slow progress filled with lots of pain and suffering along the way. It seemed that as soon as I was alone with my thoughts and no one around to motivate and inspire me, I would struggle to stay in alignment.

If only I could stay in that positive supportive environment 24/7.

Why couldn't I just do what I knew I needed to do? What was holding me back? All the while I kept feeling something inside me guiding me ... finally I thought ... there must be an easier way.

I realized that the only thing holding me back was myself, but I couldn't see, get underneath, or heal what the block was. I was blind to it. That is when I found my soul sister and mighty companion Lisa Windsor. Actually, we found each other. We became each other's coach, support, compassionate witness, accountability partner, cheerleader, and symbol of unconditional love.

We called each other every day. We were in constant contact supporting each other in the depths of our breakdowns and celebrating each other in the heights of every breakthrough. We made more progress while supporting each other than we could ever have done on our own. We were a soft place to land for each other and a voice for Truth when we couldn't hear it ourselves. We called each other on our stuff and pointed to each other's blind spots. I had never experienced such a sustainable level of support before. How powerful it was to know she was always there to support and love me no matter what. I realized we were not meant to do this on our own. I recognized the power of loving support.

I also started to see the power of healing in community when I first started teaching "Yoga for Fertility classes" at my mind-body studio in Vancouver, British Columbia. Bringing people together who are facing similar challenges was so therapeutic for them. I knew from my own struggles with fertility that it can be a very isolating experience. I would see the relief on the faces of the women as they entered the class and realized they were not alone. There was comfort in knowing that there were others who understood their fears, doubts, and challenges.

In 2011, I felt like I needed to break through a thick layer of self-sabotage. I knew I was the only one in my way and I was embracing the power of healing in community, so I created and began a twelve-week program called "Get Out of Your Own Way." I personally invited some of my clients and we began our journey together. Each week the lessons would flow through me like a gift intended for me and the participants. While I was facilitating I was integrating the lessons myself as well as helping everyone get to the root of their blocks by providing live weekly calls. It was so powerful that many participants asked if they could continue being on the weekly calls after they completed the twelve-week program. It was in that moment that the Heart Led Living community was conceived.

The weekly calls continued along with support on our private Facebook page between times. The breakthroughs were incredible and everyone, including me, was experiencing sustainable results. I would set an intention on every call to be of the highest service to the group, whether they attended the live call or tuned in to the replay.

All the while I was embracing my intuitive gift and deepening my trust and confidence in the guidance and energy that was coming through me. My intuition was getting stronger and more laser focused.

Participants were telling me how they were receiving some insight and healing from every call whether they spoke or not, whether they attended live, or listened to the replay. They loved having the personal support that prevented them from losing their footing and being able to reach out in those moments when they were being pulled down into the wormhole of fear.

My faith in healing within community grew exponentially and through my heart I gave birth to the Heart Led Living community.

I was ready to deliver exactly what everyone needed to heal at the deepest possible level.

As an intuitive coach and healer, I became a clear channel for love, healing energy, and soul insights.

Lead with Your Heart

It is not a coincidence you are holding this book and reading these words at this moment. There is something in this book that will inspire you, empower you, influence your path, and/or potentially change the course of your life. You are showing up for a divine appointment. Your heart led you here.

One of the ten principles from my book *Heart Led Living ~ When Hard Work Becomes Heart Work* is "Lead with your Heart." It teaches us to get out of our head, get into our heart, and feel our heart's YES. A true heart YES is a feeling not a thought. It is a knowing that goes beyond our mind and a feeling of expansion and Truth from deep within. A heart's YES leads us to the experiences that are meant to be on our path. Our YES for life leads us to every step in every moment that will allow us to play our part and fulfill our soul's script.

Our soul script is something we wrote before we arrived here as a human being. Imagine your soul sitting down at a board table with your soul team and determining what life lessons you are meant to learn. Imagine placing specific life experiences that will provide exactly what you need in this lifetime for the evolution of your soul. Everyone in your soul team agrees to play their part in order to support you, and you agree to play your part in their soul script as well. Our soul script is designed for our deepest healing and our greatest awakening. Some people play a part to awaken and some agree to stay asleep for most or all of their lifetime. Everyone has an integral role to play.

The authors you are about to meet felt the call and were willing to play their part. They have poured their heart and soul into their stories. They used the process of writing, editing, and putting this book together to face and overcome their fears, to heal all the hidden leftovers, to overcome self-limiting beliefs and self-sabotage, and to experience yet another miracle as they joined in love to give birth to this beautiful book.

Whether you are a seeker of Truth with a curious mind, someone who yearns for more, someone who is looking for meaning and purpose, or you are simply holding this book because someone recommended it or you just happened upon it, there is something bigger than all of us playing out, and this book is part of your divine plan to heal and awaken.

Everything that shows up on our path has meaning. We don't always discover its meaning and purpose right away. Most people find meaning and can make sense of something after they have moved through it with hindsight. If we practise "present moment hindsight" we can be open to finding meaning *during* the storm or while we are still in the depths of a specific life event. We open our minds to seeing the perfection that is playing out; we understand that if it is on our path it is purposeful, it is for our deepest healing, and it is designed to create awareness to help awaken us to another perspective for our life. We can practise present moment hindsight even in our most challenging life experiences and this fosters a deep level of peace that can carry us through the storm or challenge.

This book is divinely timed for all of humanity as all of our collective darkness is being uncovered and revealed for our deepest healing and greatest awakening. We all have a part to play. Every part is equally important. The authors in this book are courageously playing their part. Perhaps their stories will inspire you to get clearer around the part you are meant to play.

In my book *Heart Led Living ~ When Hard Work Becomes Heart Work*, I share ten principles and provide the heartwork (homework) to teach others how to use and integrate them in their everyday life classroom. The principles and tools are designed to build confidence and trust as we use our intuition as an internal GPS to guide our every decision in every moment of our life.

The Heart Led Living principles are sprinkled throughout the pages of this book and each word is infused with love and healing energy.

Here are the ten Heart Led Living principles:

1. Be willing to heal
2. Choose love
3. Hold your light
4. Take inspired action only
5. Fill your heart first
6. Be open to anything
7. Be curious

8. Be attached to nothing
9. Lead with your heart
10. Expect miracles

As I said and you will recognize, there is a reason that you are holding this book at this time. Take a deep breath and imagine your mind wide open; soften your heart. Set an intention to take what resonates with you and let your heart lead you to the gems, insights, and aha moments that are meant for you and your life. You may even be inspired to make a list that you can add to as you are reading. You can use your list to integrate these gifts into your life.

As you read this book I encourage you to make a conscious choice to use it to heal what you are meant to heal, receive the gifts of awareness, and open your heart to love. Be willing to heal, be curious, lead with your heart, be attached to nothing, be wide open to anything and, most importantly, expect miracles.

Heart hugs, Sue

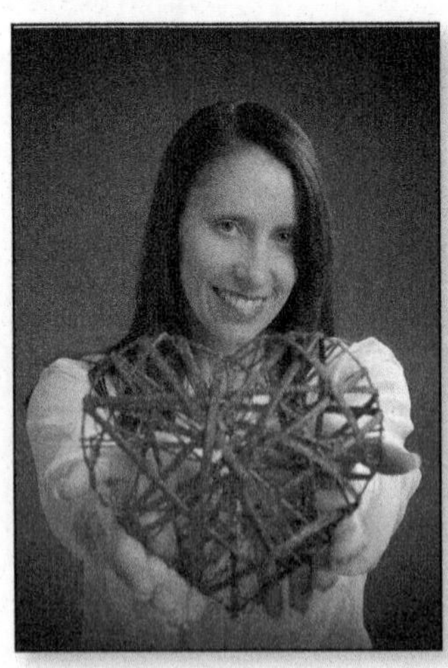

Biography for Sue Dumais, Intuitive Healer and Founder of Heart Led Living

Sue Dumais is a Heart Led Living Intuitive Coach, a best-selling author, an international speaker, and a gifted intuitive healer who helps others see the invisible, feel the intangible, and do the impossible. Sue brings the gifts of insight, awareness, and self-empowerment to her Heart Led

Living community and inspires her members to share their journey and thereby empower others through this collaborative book project.

Since 2015, Sue has been training and mentoring healers, empaths, lightworkers, and intuitive coaches to deepen their trust, build their confidence, and expand their gifts as they align with their soul's purpose. The authors in this book have all worked closely with Sue, and many have been trained through her advanced mentoring program. Their commitment and willingness to heal is palpable. They leave no stone unturned, face their fears with tremendous courage, and are dedicated to using their life as a classroom for their own deepest healing and greatest awakening.

Sue's mission is to ignite our hearts to uplift humanity and unify us in love for each other and our planet. Investing in our own healing creates a ripple effect to heal our planet. A humanitarian at heart, in 2015 Sue created the Heart Led Living Foundation to extend love and healing energy as well as emotional and financial support to empower women and girls in Kenya. One hundred percent of the royalties from this book will go to the Heart Led Living Foundation's Kenya project to empower young girls to stay in school.

Sue's previous book *Heart Led Living ~ When Hard Work Becomes Heart Work* features the ten heart led living principles that are taught to the community and in the advanced mentoring program. Sue's intuitive guidance and insights help her members awaken their innate ability to heal by trusting their intuition as they lead with their heart and discover their "YES!" for life. Learn more at heartledliving.com.

Chapter 1

Stepping out of the Darkness and into the Light

by Kimberly Shuttleworth

Stepping out of the Darkness and into the Light

by Kimberly Shuttleworth

Gifts Deep in My Core

Ever since I was a little girl, I want to say my first recollection was when I was three or four years old, I knew there was something special inside me. I had this light, this spark of energy, a flame … something unexplainable … and I could feel it deep in my core but I didn't understand it. It was merely a deep knowing almost as though God had told me or sent an angel to tell me that I had been chosen to be a lightworker. It was just a visit in one of my dreams, but it felt so real.

I remember knowing stuff before it would happen. A flash of a picture would come into my awareness or a smell or a feeling, and I would be totally taken off guard when it actually came into fruition. I could feel what others were feeling before they even said anything; this would happen automatically without any effort when I walked into a room.

One day I was playing outside; I was climbing, first a slide and then a tree. I wanted to climb up to the clouds; I wanted to go even higher, because I knew there was more out there. I wanted to converse with the angel who visited me in my dreams. I wanted to understand things better, because at that time nothing made sense to me.

It was as if this spark was always bigger than my brain could comprehend and process, and there definitely was no way I could put words to it.

This spark was my gift.

As I navigated life, there were many times I was afraid that I would lose this gift. I was afraid that it would get blown out by others and sometimes even by myself. Despite being afraid, I also found this gift overwhelming and confusing. I noticed that how I felt could change depending on other people's moods around me. It's as if I would be happy and content and, yet if I walked into a room where there was tension, I would immediately feel that and take on the energy and try to alleviate the pain for others. At such a young age, I didn't know how to handle this; I didn't know what to do or even what was happening. This was a heavy burden for a little kid.

And as much as it was normal for me, it was confusing and frustrating, not knowing or having any control over how my day would go. Would I be energized if I went to a social gathering or would I be depleted? The truth was my mood would be based on other peoples' energies in that particular moment, not on my own.

Exuberant Energy

My childhood took an unexpected turn when I entered the public school system. I had an exuberant amount of energy and I struggled to know how to manage it. I wanted so badly to fit in that I would force myself to try to be perfect so others would accept me. But it was so painful at such a young age to sit still and be "good," so to say. Internally, I instinctually really just wanted to follow my energy patterns instead of trying to fit into the school system's, but that's not how the real world works. In a seven-year-old's mind, if I fitted in and didn't get in trouble, then it was a good day. If my energy was too big and I got talked to, it was a bad day.

I remember in a primary grade, I was skipping down the hallway at school and minding my own business. In fact, I was off in space daydreaming; I was in a nice safe place in my mind and it was so wonderful. My teacher saw me and got really angry at me. I got punished. I was sent back to where I had come from and I had to re-walk the entire route "properly." Wowsers! That was so hard for me. I was choking back tears the entire time. I felt so ashamed to be me. "Come on, Kimberly. You can do better," is what I used to say to myself. And thus started the quest for perfectionism. Each time I received feedback I would feel "there is something wrong with me," which led to a core story that evolved into the "I'm not good enough" tape.

I was reminded on a daily basis that letting my inner self shine was not safe. "I need to be better at discerning when to let this light out and when to keep it hidden so that I don't get in trouble." And yet I still got teased by kids on the school bus, because as soon as I jumped off the bus I would run up our 80-metre driveway as fast as I could. It wasn't because I wanted to be home; it was just because I needed to get rid of the stored-up energy that I had been shoving down and trying to control all day long.

I felt as though I was in a catch-22—damned if I do and damned if I don't. Hopelessness was a recurring feeling during my schooling. Some days I just wished I was invisible.

Intuiting the Right Number

There was one day that I *was* seen and it just so happened to be the day I used my intuition to manifest a want. It was at the end of a school year, and the teacher was auctioning off classroom art projects to the students. One particular project was an apple tree. I have no clue now why I wanted it so badly then, but I felt as though it was to be mine. The teacher would write down a number on a piece of paper and then ask kids to guess. Whoever guessed the number first would get the item being auctioned. I really, really wanted this apple tree. Of course, I was being unique and standing off to the side a little bit, as opposed to sitting down on the mat like everyone else. I raised my hand and I wiggled around so that she would see me. I really, really, really wanted this. She chose me to go first. I was seen! Holy moly! Is this really going to be mine? So I closed my eyes really tightly and said, "… Seven." And then I waited in anticipation for her response. I can still feel how crystal clear everything felt in that moment … all the air left my lungs and she said, "Did you cheat?"

WHAT?!

An instant flow of overwhelming emotions took over my entire body. My head was racing, my heart was pounding. I clammed up inside. I struggled to find words. I managed to squeak out a small, "No," because that was my truth. But my heart crumbled, because she didn't believe me.

I was allowed to take the tree home, but all the life had been drained out of it. It went into the trash because it reminded me that when I follow my intuition and other people have a defensive position, I get hurt and embarrassed. This was another one of those days when I wished I was invisible.

I struggled in my first few years of school; first my energy and now my intuition felt as though they had betrayed me. I needed to learn better and faster how to keep these gifts hidden. I was starting to not like school because I didn't feel safe.

Shortly after these incidents took place, I was labelled with dyslexia, which in my case showed up as an auditory reading and language comprehension difficulty. I attached to this label, because it made the best explanation in my head to answer the "What is wrong with me?" question. I felt I finally had an answer. But it wasn't an answer—it was a spiritual death trap. The label actually compounded my problem of not shining my light and gave me something to hide behind to blame all my problems on.

Trying to Be Normal

Every school day was a coin toss. "Is today going to be a good day? Will I be successful at hiding my gifts and making it through the day without bringing attention to myself?"

I tried to disappear because I felt so misunderstood. I pushed myself hard to get good grades but at the expense of happiness and balance. I would work my butt off at home each night trying to fit a round peg into a square hole, always coming up short in the end, just to repeat the same cycle night after night.

As much as I wanted to stay hidden due to fear, the truth is I really wanted to be seen and understood. I wanted to be accepted, yet I was so afraid of what others would think if they knew the truth about me and the gifts I had.

All I wanted to do was fit in. "To be normal." On the outside, I looked completely normal to my friends and family … but on the inside, it was a completely different story. I was ashamed of who I was on the inside. I mean, I liked my kindness and my compassion, but I was ashamed of my gifts. So I dimmed my light as much as I could and pretended that I didn't hurt inside. By making this decision, I felt like I was in prison, shackled and shoved into a tiny room that was cold, dark, and lonely.

My internal world was a living hell. And it kept getting smaller and smaller as I got older. I turned to sports to support me and help me navigate the process.

All I wanted was to get my marks and get the eff out of Dodge.

Running and Hiding

University took me longer to get through than the average person but I did it. I received my Bachelor of Science in Human Kinetics from the University of Guelph in Ontario.

And two weeks after I finished, I got my tongue pierced and booked a ticket to go to an amazing, world-famous ski resort town in British Columbia (BC) known as Whistler. Why? Because, I just needed to run away for a bit. I needed to not feel the inner turmoil that had plagued me for twenty years. I needed to be free to experience life as far away from school and learning and the heavy feelings associated with all of that.

As I boarded the plane, I felt sure that the "real world" was going to be way different. It was going to be amazing. My intention was to go for six months to get everything out of my system, and then head back home and become the responsible person I was supposed to be.

Reality check: the real world wasn't much better. My hope bubble burst really quickly.

While I was in Whistler, I realized that everyone was running away from something, myself included. I remember clearly standing on top of the snow-covered mountain making a conscious choice: "I want to stop running." I wanted to feel different inside. I had this deep feeling inside me, "There has to be more to life than this." So I decided to set out on a journey to discover what *more* felt like and to uncover the truth inside myself.

I knew that going home to a small town and not having a car or a job or a clear direction on what I wanted to do was not how I needed to be to discover who I was and what my purpose in life was. That approach would have been a step backwards. Instead, the call of Vancouver, the big city, captured my heart. The resources, bountiful opportunities, and the closeness to nature from the mountains to the ocean appealed. It was a toss-up, but basically my decision came down to fear, the fear of not being able to shine my light in a small town. So I chose the big city.

Short-Term Relief

I started out on this self-discovery journey with high expectations and great hopes. I put a lot of money, energy, and time into "searching" for the answer. I took courses, read books, hired a declutterer, tried EMDR, life coaching, osteopathy, yoga, somato-emotional releases, counselling, tapping, meditations, crystals, essential oils, Feng Shui, and a lot of journaling and verbal processing. You name it, I tried it.

With all the searching, came a lot of aha moments. However, with each breakthrough, there was only short-term relief from the internal pain. What I realized was that some of these solutions were external in nature. At times, I wasn't actually solving the problem; I was just transferring it to a new scenario. For example, I left a part-time job thinking it was the job that was my problem, only to find myself in the same predicament three months later in a new part-time job. Nothing changes if nothing changes. It was easier to change my external physical surroundings than it was to change my internal perspective.

From Thinking to Breathing

Despite the "hard work" I put into searching for the answers, what I didn't realize at the time was that the key to healing and transforming my life was inside me. I didn't need to look externally for the answers anymore; I just needed to go directly to my heart and bypass my mind. And this scared the heck out of me. But I did it anyway. Slowly, as I had more and more success going inwards, I realized that this is where I needed to hang out more and more. I would bounce back and forth between trying to heal internally and externally. One of the tools that would support me to stay inward was my breath.

Looking back at all the money I spent on books and courses, I realize still to this day that the best tool of all time is my breath. Breathing with awareness brings insight and calmness. My breath allows me to slow down and start listening to my heart, to hear what is happening internally.

I realized that there was a lot of chatter up there in my head. The "shoulds," the expectations of myself and others, the "I'm not good enough" tape, the "you suck, you're going to make a mistake" message. When I used my breath to stop all the tapes from playing out, I started to realize that there was another voice hanging out with my ego. It was Spirit's voice. It took many hours and much dedication to learn how to decipher between ego and Spirit. Sometimes, the ego would disguise himself as love, which was tricky to catch. But slowly over time, I was able to discern between love and fear.

In the past, a noticeable theme would arise for me that, each time I needed to go deeper, I would have physical pain. In the beginning, I would miss this cue from the Universe, because I used to use exercise to avoid my feelings. Exercise was my go-to tool to survive university. When I played varsity sports, the philosophy was "no pain no gain." So it makes sense that I missed this cue. Since embarking on the healing journey, pain in my body changed its meaning. I used to avoid doing my internal work and now I wasn't able to because the pain in my body would intensify really quickly and become too great to bear. The pain in my body was merely a sign for me that I needed to stop and go inwards.

I found it interesting that when there was a calling to go deeper, to take a step, to jump, the Universe would provide me with the opportunity to do so. If I missed the opportunity by not taking action, somehow the opportunity would come back around or one similar would appear.

Rhodes Wellness College

Spirit guided me to interview to attend Rhodes Wellness College in Vancouver and learn life coaching. And ego talked me out of it: "You can't do school. It was so hard the first time around. How are you going to pay your bills? This is crazy."

I kept the brochure in my files and let the idea of becoming a life coach go for the meantime. Three years later, a friend went to the school and immediately thought it would be a good fit for me as I was still searching for that perfect job. When I went to have the interview, I didn't even realize that I had been there before, until I stepped into the elevator and a feeling of déjà vu overcame me. After the interview, I knew right away that was where I needed to be.

Going back to school was part of my healing process. I was able to unwind from the trauma I experienced being labelled with a learning disability. I was drawn to choose a school where students learn experientially. I didn't have to sit and read a textbook and regurgitate the information. Through my own experiences and those of others, I learned the lessons that were being taught. I excel in this type of learning. What you put into the program is what you get out of it. So the deeper I went into my wounds, the greater the healing that occurred.

When I graduated from Rhodes Wellness College, I received both my Wellness Counselling Diploma and my Life Skills Coach Certificate.

It was in the moment of shifting my personal training business to include a phone coaching wellness component that I felt "on purpose" for the first time. I mean, I was good at personal training, but I was in my zone of genius (as Gay Hendricks explains in *The Big Leap*) when I was coaching on the phone. The phone provided me with a safe place to be able to listen with my inner ear and tune in for what messages I was to give.

Some Big Life Changes

I put my search for a career on hold when my personal life took priority. For the next two years, my boyfriend and I became engaged, we bought a house, and I birthed two children. These were a lot of big life changes. As much as each individual moment was filled with joy and excitement, together they took a toll on me. My body ached, my mind felt like scrambled eggs, and my heart was breaking. As I was trying my hardest to hold it all together, I realized I really had no control over anything and I was feeling overwhelmed and confused. I didn't know which way to turn.

I vividly remember one day sitting on the bed doing diaper duty and praying for an extra-long afternoon nap when a message came clearly that I was not to go back to work—I was needed at home. Unfortunately, the financial option in my life at that current moment made more noise. I made the conscious decision to go against my heart and go back to work, because it made financial sense and I didn't trust that we would be okay otherwise.

My productivity went down in all areas of my life. I hated being away from the kids when I was going to a job that was not fulfilling me anymore. My life felt torturous. I tried externally changing my shifts at work to better suit me—again, this was an external solution for an internal problem. The Universe provided again, not once but twice.

When my son was sixteen months old, he had a health scare and needed medical intervention. Navigating this became a top priority, so I took some time off work and never went back. My partner was emotionally unable to support me or my son through this bump in the road. So I navigated the pathway on my own. I needed to dig deep emotionally, but this experience provided me with the knowledge and strength and courage that I am capable, resourceful, and strong. At the time, I didn't realize how valuable this experience would be.

Shortly thereafter, the Universe provided the opportunity

for me to leave my relationship. Becoming a single mom was my biggest fear playing itself out. Yet everything inside me said, "Do it." Now when the Universe says jump and you jump, things tend to happen quickly. The next message I received was, "Move to Ontario." What! This is insane. I was already leaving my relationship; now you are saying leave my home, my part-time job, and everything I have known for the past fifteen years?

I left BC with sixty dollars in my pocket and I was literally scared out of my mind feeling an immense pressure to not screw it up. I was working on blind faith, because I literally had no clue what I was doing. The only things I had were myself, my two kids, and this internal knowing, this flame inside me. The immense pressure I felt that I couldn't screw up weighed on my shoulders. I felt as though I had failed. Not because my relationship was over. Not because of the lack of money in my bank account. But because I still hadn't been able to shine my light. I hadn't even come close to it. What came next was a rollercoaster ride of ups and downs full of aha moments and heartbreak. I was working on the deep faith that the Universe would catch me and provide. And it did, every step of the way.

Starting over the second time around was a little more scary because I was also responsible for two beautiful, young, innocent boys who deserve a really great life. They became my motivation to continue moving forward. I prayed long and hard for a miracle for this uphill climb. I had my faith in the Universe. I had my internal strength and courage. I had my tools. When I thought about the past I was sad; when I thought about the future I was anxious. The present moment was the only place I could find peace and calm.

The Heart Led Living Community

During my first year back in Ontario, I sought out support, both professionally and personally. I joined the Heart Led Living (HLL) community, which provided me with the foundation of healing from my past and illuminating my future. I worked the tools daily. I got out of my head, which is where my ego is. And I fully immersed myself to live my life at my heart. I showed up every week for guidance from my mentor Sue Dumais. I wasn't able to hear all the guidance clearly, so I needed someone who is a clear and open channel to decipher it for me. My confidence grew week by week.

For two years I yo-yoed back and forth from my head to my heart. I could never figure it out in my head. So I needed to constantly be pointed back to my heart. And I learned to trust that the answers are always there. Each failure as judged by the outside world was an internal success to me.

I used these opportunities to propel me forward in my healing process. I cleared out emotional baggage; I unwound from the mental and the physical body. Spiritually and energetically, I cleansed. My curriculum was my classroom of life. I would bring my triggers from my life to each call so that I could get to the root cause and pull it. I showed up week after week wanting more, going deeper. It was as if healing was my jam. I couldn't get enough of it.

As I started to trust myself and gain confidence in my ability to channel messages, I slowly started taking down my blocks to my heart. And each time I removed a block, I was making the choice for peace. Peace from the chaos inside me. Now that I had created space around my heart and shifted my internal world, my confidence and skills continued to grow. I was so proud of the depths to which I was healing. I felt that I could breathe again.

I Came to a Complete Stop

Just when I thought I was going to step out and spread my wings, the Universe once again had other plans. Two years to the exact day that I had moved to Ontario, I slipped on ice and fell, breaking my ankle in three places. I came to a complete stop. I was confused because of all the growth and progress I had made internally. This put a halt on the external part of the equation. Little ego Kimberly wanted to get a job, start a career, and bring her bank account out of the red. However, I was meant to stay on the couch and go deeper.

Something miraculous happened during the recovery of my ankle. I received "a heart yes" to sign up for HLL's intuitive healing and coaching program. I kept this quiet for almost two years. I was afraid to talk about it, to share it with family and friends at first. Seeing that I had had a gift of feeling other people's energy from a young age, I decided to tap back into this and see where it went. I was being trained by intuitive healer Sue Dumais to trust my intuition so that I could become a clear and open channel for others to get messages for facilitating their healing. With every fibre in my body, I was clear that I am meant to be a healer. How this looked, I had no clue as I entered into this vortex of healing.

Each day I would show up and move toward the light, because that is where the answers lie. The truth lies not in the darkness but in the light. The more light I shone on myself, the more complete or whole I felt. Don't get me wrong; I wanted to quit and leave the program on numerous occasions. However, in each moment, I chose love; I chose to look into the dark corners inside me, and expose the dense thick energy that was holding me back from shining my light for all those years.

Shining My Light Both In and Out

I did not feel the rewards of this hard personal journey until just recently when everything finally clicked and I was guided to start shining my light externally.

My life is so different now. How I parent, how I show up in the world, what I say yes to. I have gotten out of my head and I live my life from my heart.

I follow my energy as one of my signposts. I tap into my intuition for information. I practise the tools daily for myself and with my children.

My connections are rich and deep, and my circles are small and sacred.

My life is directed by a higher power and my only job is to follow the guidance.

I feel authentic and alive.

Looking back I can see how perfection played out. I saw how leaving Ontario for BC was purposeful. I see how leaving BC to come back to Ontario was purposeful. I especially see how breaking an ankle was purposeful (even though I could have done without that lesson being so harsh). It was all playing out for my benefit. I finally found my way home to a place deep inside myself. And not only did I find it, I was able to find the strength and courage to light it up. I overcame my biggest fears and struggles. The pain of actually trying to stay hidden was my catalyst down this road of healing and enlightenment. It woke me up.

What they say is true—your biggest obstacles become your greatest gifts.

I'm not normal and I'm never going to fit in and for the first time in my life that's okay. Actually, it's great, to be honest. I was never meant to fit into a box; that was out of fear. I was meant to shine brightly, to be a clear and open channel for those who I am meant to help. I have a deep calling to support others to heal. And I can do this as an intuitive healer and coach.

I was called at a young age to be a lightworker, but I didn't understand it and how to use this gift to help others, so it was easier to turn my back on it. Now my job is simple—I shine my light. And this supports others along their healing journey. Some are drawn toward me and others run the other way for fear of their darkness. I have been there; I get it.

I choose love each and every day, knowing that my higher power has my back.

Namaste, Kimberly

Tips

1. Breathe deeply—and follow the breath inwards.
2. Trust the process—even when it doesn't make sense.
3. Follow your heart—there's no wrong answer or turn.

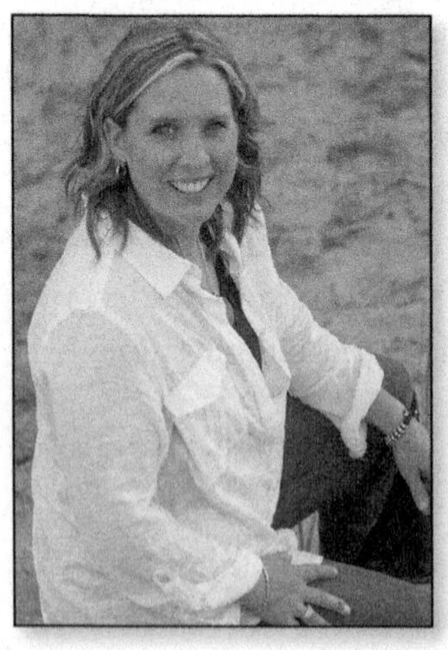

Author Biography for Kimberly Shuttleworth, BSc, HK, Wellness Counsellor, Life Skills Coach, Heart Led Living Intuitive Healer and Coach, Sacred Gifts Certified Guide

Kimberly Shuttleworth was a free-spirited, energetic, alive, talkative, doing cartwheels every chance she got kinda kid who loved playing and had a zest for life.

That all changed when she entered the public school system. She struggled to dial down her energy, personality, and creativity all in the hope of conforming to the status quo. This is when she first learned that she needed to dim her light to fit in and not be found out.

During her time in the educational system, Kimberly lost confidence in her ability to trust her intuition. It was evident right away that she learned differently; she was labelled with dyslexia. Self-doubt started to rent a lot of space in her head. Her internal struggle was masked by an external smile to pretend all was well. She managed to find some relief from the frustration of feeling different and unique through sports and physical activity.

At a young age, Kimberly noticed she was affected by what was on the news or if she walked into a room and there was tension. It was as if she could feel into the pain and suffering of others. As she learned more about energy, she struggled with this gift because it confused her. She thought there was something wrong with her as she started to see how a person's body language, their words, and their energy were each communicating something completely different. Kimberly found it very exhausting and hard to navigate social settings at times. She felt as though society was giving her the message that there was "something wrong with her" again, so she pushed her empathy away and tried to hide this gift.

Struggling to hide her gifts became her new normal, which led to her life becoming really hard and painful until life circumstances forced her to make a choice.

Kimberly has turned her life around 180 degrees. In the past five years, she has gone from struggling and hiding in silence to embracing her gifts and shining brightly. She joined the Heart Led Living (HLL) community and was introduced to its principles, which she started using daily. As she learned to embrace her gifts, her intuition began to flourish. She was always drawn to explore alternative holistic healing, and quickly realized that she is a lightworker. She enrolled in both the intuitive coaching and advanced mentoring programs through HLL and was able to fine tune her gifts as an intuitive healer and coach.

Once Kimberly got out of her own way and found the courage to step outside the "normal box" that she had tried to stuff herself into, she was able to make a conscious choice to spread her wings. She now lives a full expression of herself, embracing her gifts and shining her light as an intuitive energy worker. She resides in Ontario with her two young sons, where they all practise the HLL principles. She works as an intuitive healer and coach while supporting people to discover their sacred gifts.

You can reach Kimberly and learn more about her offerings at heartledliving.com/our-coaches/Kimberly-Shuttleworth/.

Chapter 2

The Little Girl with the Big Secret

by Kelly Van Unen

The Little Girl with the Big Secret

by Kelly Van Unen

Not Trusting Anyone

To some people, the idea of keeping a secret for forty years may not be such a big deal. To my four-year-old self, it was a really BIG secret; I could tell NOBODY.

Deep down within, I knew it was wrong and so instead of blossoming into a flowering kindergartner, I dove deep into my shell, full of fear, shame, and sadness, not trusting anyone and especially those with an energy that felt unsafe.

I failed kindergarten, yes. Who fails kindergarten? I wouldn't speak at school or play with others. It was as though I was frozen, unable to move. My teacher thought I was shy and needed more time to develop. Luckily, my parents did not see this side of me at home and so I went on to grade 1.

For years, I feared other people's homes and I daydreamed in class, leaving me with low marks, a necessity for learning assistance, and a growing identity of thinking I was dumb.

I didn't want to grow up! I had an internal sadness that attached to my every cell. The only time I felt really safe was in my own space, playing with my Barbies or playing make belief, pretending to be a teacher. I would play behind furniture in order to hide from others who might interrupt my inner world. I played small in every way so that I felt safe. I floated through life pretending everything was fine and not knowing why I felt so many fears. In high school, I began to have more friends, which became more of a focus. Still, I felt I really wasn't good at anything. "Average" became me.

Conversations with God

I started to come out of my shell when I was sixteen. Surrounding me were men who dominated. They were intense, judgmental, and seemed to be able to speak their minds. I never really felt I could properly communicate with them. Around this time, I completely engulfed myself in a relationship with a boy for four years. This taught me more about myself than I knew before. This boy was someone who distracted me from the outside world and got me away from my home. I felt safe when it was just the two of us. I could just be my small self, and follow his guidance and stronger aura. This was an interesting time as my whole heart dove into his heart. I felt his actions affecting me in a way that encompassed me, whether they were good or not so good.

Two years into the relationship, I felt like a robot—I was so emotionally attached. Something happened that made me realize this and I started to close off even more to others, but at the same time, I opened up to what I called "God." I felt I had nobody else to talk to about my feelings so I had conversations with God. I asked for strength, courage, and direction. Slowly over the last two years of this relationship, my mindset started to change. I started doing things that I felt were good for me. I started to call my own shots. I began to gain more independence, courage, and direction in my life. I knew that this four-year relationship with my best friend at the time needed to end. It no longer served either one of us and we had to move on. It was the hardest decision, but I knew in my heart it was the right thing to do. When there is a clear knowing, it is much easier to make decisions that change the course of one's life.

My father was an entrepreneur and he suggested I should have a job by the age of fourteen. He taught me how to be successful in his terms, through time-management, list writing, goal-setting, and so on. I dove into this and listened to what he had to say because I knew that he was successful, and I wanted to be successful too.

Living in Two Worlds

When I was twenty-three, my then-fiancé (he is now my husband) and I started our own interior design business. I had worked for two design firms in prior years and went to design school in the evenings. I was living life the way everyone thinks it should be lived: hard work, long hours, focusing on doing a job to perfection, and working my way up the ladder. I was living paycheque to paycheque, but feeling as though I was accomplishing something.

I loved what I was doing and we became very busy. At this time in my life, I really felt that my life was picture perfect! I had the perfect upbringing, the perfect parents, the now-perfect husband with his perfect family, along with my perfect career. Now, my secret was so deep within that I just kept piling life on top of it. If everything looks perfect from the outside, then it must be perfect inside.

In some ways, you could say that I was living in two worlds. My outer world was not necessarily in alignment with my inside world. When I feel back to my twenties, I realize I was a driven person who wanted success and wanted to be recognized as successful. This came at a cost to my body first; I was diagnosed with irritable bowel syndrome.

Also, I developed a pattern of holding in all my feelings, thoughts, and emotions for as long as I could until I could do so no longer. My husband said to me one day, "Kelly, why do you hold everything in for months until you explode?"

Months of "STUFF" would fly out of my mouth with tears and shame. Frustration and anger were synonymous. He is the type of person who says how he feels in the moment. Thank God! He has been one of my communication teachers in my life.

Then we became parents of two boys, three years apart. I grew up in a family that believed in physical and verbal discipline and in the seventies and eighties; this was probably not unusual. It wasn't until I had my own children that I realized how badly I felt when I spanked my kids for the first time. Yes, it took more than once to realize that I was out of control.

I had never been taught to breathe in a moment of despair or to calm myself in order to make a decision that was in alignment with me and my child. We all have these moments when all we want to do is scream, but what if we just feel what is happening? It was a time in my life when I could only acknowledge my feelings once I could not hold them in any longer. This often resulted in tears and discussions with my husband, and it released much of the built-up energy, but it never touched the issues deep within. Being vulnerable was dangerous to me. I needed to feel in control of my life and in order to do that, I kept my heart safe and somewhat closed.

Asking Big Questions

I was forty when my close friend Wendy died. She was my fifth friend to die of cancer in five years, all but one of them leaving behind their young children. This experience stopped me in my tracks. I wanted my life to slow down so I could truly live, so I could feel into my life, so I could feel free.

My curiosity was asking BIG questions: Why are we here? What is my true purpose? How can I make my life more fulfilling?

I yearned for freedom, flow, less anxiety, less busyness, and more meaning in my life. I wanted to get off the treadmill. I felt I needed to spend more quality time with people, the universe, and my connection to it all. My husband was also ready for a change. We started with our day-to-day life. Instead of selling our business of sixteen years, we decided to give it away. We gave all our clients to another interior designer who would take care of our customers. Now, ten years later, she still is taking good care of them, just as we knew she would.

I took the freed-up time to dive into myself and that is when the puzzle pieces started to link together.

Somehow, I had forgotten my secret from the time it happened until I was forty years old. It disappeared deep within me. It was as though an earthquake had occurred and all the rubble had fallen on top of the secret, burying it; but I was still alive. The patterns of shame, fear, anxiety, and sadness continued.

For most of my life, I believed that if I did something for myself, that was selfish. I would feel guilty and unable to enjoy the moment. I was really good at giving and saying yes to other people, but I was not so good at receiving. I was a people pleaser. I have never felt comfortable in tense situations, so I have tried to avoid all confrontations and uncomfortable situations. The fear that rose in me when my brothers or I were disciplined was extreme. All I wanted to do was keep the peace. One of my brothers decided that he was going to rebel, so I found myself praying for quiet and peace in my home. It was difficult to find the love in all of this fear and anger. I craved loving moments and wondered why there weren't more of those moments. I now realize that I felt the unhappiness for everyone in my family and my circle of friends. I would not allow myself to feel beyond their emotional wellbeing, because I didn't feel good about the idea of feeling better than them. The combination of hiding myself most of the time and feeling others' emotions made me feel as though I were in a constant flux. My happiness depended on the behaviour and mood of whoever surrounded me at the time.

On her website, Oprah says, "No experience is ever wasted. Everything has meaning."

I give credit to all my experiences moving me toward shifting and starting my movement inward! My healing journey began when my secret started to reveal itself.

As much as I seemed like a shy person to the outside world, I was not as shy at home. I was always a curious person, with a childhood family nickname of Nosy Rosy. I wanted to know about the truth of what was going on with everyone in the family. I wanted to be included in my parents' conversations. I felt a need to know because I could feel the emotions behind the silence. I was always fascinated with people's interactions and how their energies would work or not work with each other.

As a teenager, I dove into the unknown—Ouija boards, tarot cards, psychics. I was more fearful of someone finding out that I liked these things than I was afraid of taking part in them. I took solace in the unknown including, in all of this, God. I felt very alone in my world. I grew up in the church and felt a deep connection with what I then called God and now call Spirit. Over the years I have been inconsistent with my connection with Spirit; however, my feeling of Spirit has never diminished. Spirit has been my true companion, the miracle in my life, and my saving grace. I came to realize that my relationship with Spirit was much more than I had at my church and with the people in my church. I needed to strip away all the judgment and fear in order to feel what I knew to be Spirit. I now feel that I am one with Spirit.

During my exploration of my connection to something much bigger than myself yet part of me, I have had many teachers show up. All the miracle workers I came across have one common denominator: they all believe in their own connection to something spiritual, a universal energy. The more time I spent with them, the more I felt at home. Being in their presence allowed me to expand my own spiritual awareness without feeling judged or manipulated. It allowed me to open up for healing.

Inner Child Meditation

One of my mentors, Sue Dumais, invited me to a weekend retreat she was hosting at her home outside Vancouver. At that point I had been working with her for a few years, but mostly just on her weekly group phone calls and the odd one-day workshop. I knew I was to attend this retreat, but it was for a reason that I would never have imagined.

I don't recollect much of the weekend as I became so all-consumed with my forty-year secret that revealed itself in an inner child guided meditation. After the meditation, we were asked to express our feelings around what had come through. I began to make myself small, pulling my legs to my chest and allowing my head to fall to my knees. Tears began to engulf my eyes and then my face. My breath got short and I did not hear what any of the others were saying. Instead, my head was saying, "Don't tell" and my heart was saying, "It is time to tell someone." I was forty-four. Nobody knew, not even my husband of twenty years.

I felt I could trust Sue and the other women, so I blurted it out. "I had a sexual altercation with a man when I was four." With my body shaking, I also said, "You are the first to know." That was the first layer of my healing around my inner child, but not my last.

I later found out that four out of the five women at the retreat had been sexually abused as children. We shared some stories and felt each other's pain. I left that conversation feeling as though there was hope and there was a gem among the rubble. It was the beginning of removing one piece of stone at a time in order to heal my secret.

The next boulder I had to overcome was telling my husband. I left the retreat knowing this had to happen. I felt sick to my stomach for two days and could no longer keep it from him. The tears were running down my face that evening and I could barely get a word out. He is one of the kindest people I have ever met and I felt so grateful that he was so patient and loving to me, when I finally blurted it out. I felt great relief and quite a bit of closure.

I still had more rubble to overcome. The next was to forgive the man. Surprisingly, this has been the easiest part. I have the ability to see good in all people and this has served me well in my life.

To me, everyone is born as an innocent baby and then they become products of their environment, good and bad. People do things to people depending on how they are feeling internally. If you are feeling pain, often you want others to feel pain or you want them to see your pain. When we do things to others, we are searching to feel good. No matter whether we are doing something good or bad, what we do, think, and feel manifests and attracts more of the same thing. When we change our thoughts, we change what we attract.

We give life to what we energize. It is difficult to remove ourself from something that makes us feel good in the moment but bad afterwards. Quite often, we call that an addiction. Whether it is a drug, alcohol, sex, or food addiction, it is masking the deep-seated problem of the human being. It is filling in the space that feels empty or it is piling stuff on top so we can't feel the pain. This prevents healing. I piled life on top of life so I could not feel anything unless I wanted to. I needed the control over my life. I look back and wonder why I didn't turn to drugs, alcohol, or food. I say fear saved my life here. I felt if I let my guard down and wasn't in control that something bad could happen again. I dabbled with alcohol, but I never got to the point where I wasn't conscious of my surroundings. Also, because I was a natural observer of life, I saw what alcohol and drugs did to people and I wanted to avoid that.

Beyond Sleepwalking

We become comfortable with our life as we know it. We close

ourselves off from possibilities that are outside our comfort zone. We fear the unknown and stay stuck in the mundane. A few years ago, one day after an inspiring talk I gave on living your best life, a seventeen-year-old student was leaving when she looked into my eyes and said, "We are kinda sleepwalking through life."

I said to her, "You are so right!"

She had realized something that most people take their entire lives to understand. I could so relate to this young woman's analogy. Why do we sleepwalk through life? Why do we pile rubble on top of things we don't want to look at? Why do we mask our problems with addiction? This isn't a minor issue; this is a global issue. I believe we have a choice of how we live on this planet.

For myself, I didn't start to wake up until I was forty. I just lived the life that I thought I was supposed to live, the life that I thought looked like the right way. I never felt calm or at peace. I was always on edge. Playing small. This is not to say I still don't have those feelings anymore. I am just more aware of them and know how to work through them. I accept them as gifts, because they bring new self-awareness and awareness of my surroundings as well as my relationships.

Some people call what I had a mid-life crisis; some call it an awakening; some call it just a change. It seems as though, once we reach mid-life, we begin to wake up to the fact that we may have taken on traits that simply aren't in alignment with who we are. Quite likely, these belong to our parents, our culture, our religion, our routines, and they become our habits.

Also, I am aware that when we come into this life we take years to learn things and then we come to realize that much of what we learned we must undo in order to be our authentic self. To be free! To feel connected to something bigger than just ourselves; a connection to LIFE here on earth and beyond.

I have found within myself the power to forgive, heal, and grow from my life experiences and I have learned how to raise my own vibration. I have given myself permission to feel into my emotions and heal all that I need to heal. I see my strength and courage, and I have truly started to live the life I deserve and the life I want, finding happiness in spite of my past.

Raise Your Vibration

No matter your past, you can always change the now.

I can help you to go inward and raise your vibration with the following tools that help me every day to connect with myself.

Awareness

Awareness is where we can start. We begin feeling our emotions ("emotion" is energy in motion) instead of covering them up and storing them within. We listen and ask what we can do to unblock this energy.

Just Breathe

Releasing unwanted energy by just breathing. Breath is the key. When I am upset with myself, my boys, my students, or my friends, the first thing out of my mouth is "Just breathe." Listen to your breath. By listening to our breath, we get out of our head. We can't listen to our breath and our thoughts at the same time. Our breath is always with us so it doesn't matter where you are in the moment. Even in class, in meetings, or in a moment of despair, we can always listen to our breath.

Be Mindful

Setting an intention to release the discomfort, pain, or thoughts that no longer serve you is important. You can do this by being mindful, starting to be aware of your thoughts and feelings. We have the capacity to change our thoughts at any time. I did this for the longest time and it's helpful on the surface, but it doesn't release the long-term effects of past negative experiences. They are often so deep that you need to peel off the layers of emotions surrounding them. You are required to feel each layer of emotion by intentionally releasing it through tears, language, feeling in the body, and/or through writing. Use anything to get it out. Think about it: Why do we feel so good after we have a good cry? Our society is taught that crying is a sign of weakness, especially for men. We need to look at this differently. Crying is a sign that we are willing to be vulnerable and vulnerability gives us permission to show the world who we truly are; it is a strength that shows courage. Vulnerability brings out your authenticity and reveals your truth and realness!

Love Yourself

Focus on your personal strengths instead of your weaknesses. We have a tendency to be hard on ourselves. We need to love ourselves. We can only give out as much love as we have for ourselves.

Have Gratitude

Have gratitude for the good stuff in your life. In our culture, it seems easier to focus on what we don't have or the ugly parts of our bodies instead of what we do have and the beauty in us. When you actually write a list of the things in your life you are grateful for, it changes everything and places you in positive observation. This helps to raise your vibration. You can actually feel the energy change.

Accept with Trust

Accept what is and let go of the results. Trust that the universe is giving you exactly what you need in order to fulfill your life's purpose. Difficult times help us to grow and expand our consciousness and awareness. Trust contributes a feeling of wellbeing; a feeling of "I've got this"; a feeling that each of us is not alone; a feeling of confidence; and a feeling of "I'm on the right path." It is a contributor not only for ourselves, but for the growth of our universe.

Drop into the Heart

We need to start to unite, communicate, and begin to make decisions from the heart rather than the mind. The heart knows BEST. The mind is to help facilitate what the heart is telling us. When we drop into the heart, we remove any ego that wants to make the decision for us. Also, we remove what the outside world has to say about it. Again, it's a feeling, like falling in love; it is inside you, not outside you.

Meditate to Connect with Source Energy

So, how do we connect with our heart, which is peace, flow, Spirit, love, and compassion? All the things we crave as humans. Meditation is one avenue for connecting. I think this is an incredible tool and moving toward this is definitely beneficial. This practice along with yoga has been very helpful for me; however, I think many people have a really hard time jumping into the practice of meditation and sustaining it.

There is another way to connect us with source energy and the universe in our everyday life and that is to feel for a specific energy. Some people give this energy different names—God, Allah, Buddha. I explain it as an energy of love. It is a feeling like no other. It is a feeling like someone is looking out for you at all times. Our truth, authenticity, love, and compassion come from this place. I call it Spirit. How can we tap into this feeling more often? By listening. Listen to that little voice inside you, it is ALWAYS right! It is your intuition; it is the truth! It is about believing in yourself enough to hear your desires and dreams and know your worthiness.

Discover Your Possibilities

I want you to discover the possibilities that live within you. I want you to stand for what you believe in and search for your truth. This has very little to do with knowledge and everything to do with awareness. Awareness of yourself, your needs, your values, your connections, your relationships, and your meaning.

There is a reason why you are reading this book and you have read this chapter. I encourage you to ask yourself why. What has drawn you toward certain parts and what parts have triggered you? In connecting yourself with these stories, you allow your heart to open up. Give yourself some quiet time to journal your thoughts. You can only be to others what you are to yourself. Give yourself the gift of getting to know your authentic self. It is your gift to the world!

Warm heart, Kelly

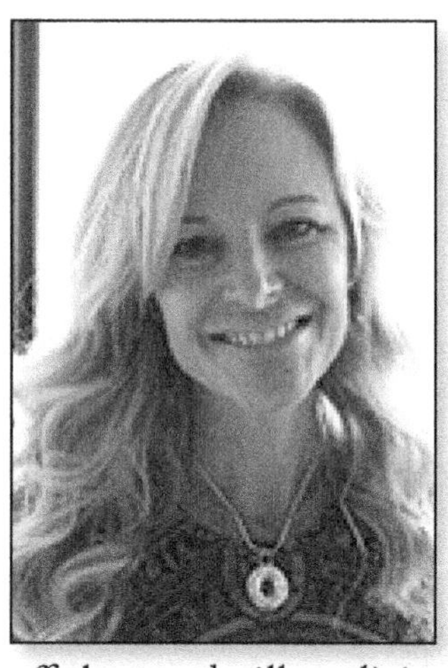

Author Biography for Kelly Van Unen, Inside Out Life Consultant

Raised in Vancouver, Canada, Kelly Van Unen studied interior design and, at the ages of twenty-two and twenty-four, she and her husband started their own interior design business. The business was successful for sixteen years when they decided to give it away and get off the treadmill, realizing they wanted more out of life than just business success. Being a mother of two boys has helped Kelly to focus on what is important in her life: communication, love, and compassion. Her volunteer work with her family's charity, Universal Outreach Foundation, has provided her with a whole new way of thinking and opened doors to the reality of life globally.

Since 2010, Kelly has studied in the Heart Led Living community with Sue Dumais, a master spiritual teacher. Having experienced personal healings of all sorts, Kelly is healing her past, present, and future, and connecting her mind, body, and soul. As a healing facilitator, Kelly is empowering the local youth of today to connect with themselves in ways that go beyond just knowledge. Her combination of passion and expertise allows her to guide her students to new levels of success in their personal growth, strengths, and wellbeing by focusing on their inner awareness.

Through her own growth, experiences, and studies, Kelly is on a mission to make it possible for people to live from the inside out, leading their life with confidence, good health, and a sense of meaning and purpose that is authentic to them. To learn more about Kelly and her offerings, visit insideoutlife.ca.

Chapter 3

Choosing Faith Over Fear

by Kent Smith

Choosing Faith over Fear

by Kent Smith

A Dysfunctional Family

Free agency is a gift given to every individual. This life is just a stage where we practise this gift. Continual choices between light and dark, good and evil are placed before each of us. We gain experience through the consequences of our choices as well as those of others. These experiences are received through our bodies. We are free to choose anything but there are always consequences attached to the choices we make. The experiences we have may be good, bad, ugly, horrific, absurd, or just plain stupid. Whatever the type of experience, they all affect, shape, and refine us. They create our personal foundation and directly influence our behaviours, perspectives, and motivations.

It's a universal truth that each of us receives our physical body through the union of a man and a woman. Our eternal spirits come into these lovely little temples and they're the vehicle of our eternal progression. We are all born innocent, pure, and clean. We fulfill our potential as infants and children as we grow, but we really don't know any differently. We are sponges that absorb patterns and knowledge from the family we're sent to. We learn and are conditioned to choose each day what we do, how we feel, and who we become.

I was born to a set of earthly parents who were brought together out of their passions but who really weren't compatible. I am grateful for their union and the gift of my body. I honour the sacrifice of the woman who bore me, but I don't recollect much of their time together. All I remember are vignettes in my maternal grandmother's house when they were going through their divorce. Going forward, I was a pawn, and my biological father had little to no access to me while I was growing up.

My mother remarried when I was four years old. This was like going from the frying pan into the fire. It was difficult all of a sudden to have three older step siblings and another dad in the house. We each had emotional baggage and became a dysfunctional family unit right out of the gate. Despite the chaos and drama that are trademarks of every alcoholic home, I received enough of the basic necessities. I had food, clothing, and shelter. There was clean air and clean water. I went to school and I was blessed to get an education. There were no wars, natural disasters, or external calamities threatening my life that I remember. Sometimes, it was pointed out to me that I was selfish, and that many of the world's children were deprived of these basics. I never understood how I could be guilty or responsible for these facts. Such statements felt threatening and so, as a child, it was easy to convince myself that what I had was enough. I always felt I was different from others. I was easily overwhelmed and felt a lot of separation anxiety. I always had a hard time feeling worthy to receive any sort of good thing. I just felt that I simply didn't deserve it.

The Price of Admission

In elementary school, I wanted to be older, because I believed that at a certain age life would start and I would be someone different. Sometimes, through middle school and high school, I would just sit and observe those around me. I never fit in. I was a chameleon. I had acquaintances in the various groups. I knew people who were athletes, artists, musicians, the mechanically inclined, the academics, the partyers, and the stoners. I had acquaintances in all these groups and so I would change my language and focus to relate to them. I didn't know who I was. I didn't know what I was. I was afraid to be seen. I was afraid to be heard. I was afraid to stand up for anything. I was afraid to let anyone in. All I really wanted was acceptance and to feel that I wasn't alone. But I wasn't willing to pay the price of admission—it seemed too much to be part of any one of these groups.

When I started working in the summers and on weekends, I continued to observe those around me. I worked in a sawmill making good money for an eighteen-year-old at the time. I would listen on my work breaks to what the other guys would be talking about or what got them excited. The majority of them would talk about the next thing they were going to buy. Most were broke, always living paycheque to paycheque. Others were living for the next party, for how much they were going to drink, for who they were lusting after or having sex with.

Whatever their focus and pursuit—the party, the sex, the car, the truck, the boat, the vacation—I would look, listen, and try it on and it always felt empty and hollow. It just didn't seem right or full or complete. Something was missing but I didn't know what. I would internally ask myself: "Is this the point? Is this the epitome of living? Is this what it means to be an adult?" It seemed that the purpose of life was empty and futile.

Listening and associating with my coworkers at times made me wonder if I was crazy. They seemed happy with their latest debauchery, their latest toy, or their latest pursuit. I found myself repeating the same old pattern in my life. I felt unsafe. I was unwilling to do whatever it would take to be accepted by them. I seemed doomed to be terminally unique and the odd one out, living a life of quiet desperation. I always wanted to feel like part of the group, but I was never willing to go all in and pay the price of admission.

Once I Get a Degree

I had enough sense to realize that the power of association is very real. We each tend to find our circle of associates in our own personal comfort zone. I saw other schoolmates succumb to the lifestyle modelled at the mill. All I knew was that I didn't want to become like those around me. I know that sounds judgmental but, even if all you have is negative motivation, it's still a force for change. This fueled my decision to go to university. I convinced myself that by completing a university degree something would change in my life. I would arrive and somehow my life would just be better.

Chasing illusions kept me from being present in the present moment. I could easily lose minutes, hours, days, weeks, and even months focused on some future event. Along with chasing illusions of the future, I also spent a great deal of time focused on things of the past. I would get stuck in analysis paralysis and fantasies of vengeance or retribution for real or perceived wrongs. This was my modus operandi and it worked well. It kept me out of touch with the reality of my life experiences.

When I started university it became clear very quickly that I was not like my peers. In my first year, I saw how I couldn't function like others. I couldn't learn as fast or retain as much. I just couldn't do it. I simply wasn't ready. I wasn't at ease with myself. I found it hard to talk to others, to laugh, and even to smile. Naturally I started judging myself even more because I couldn't do the same things my friends were doing. I couldn't study. I couldn't work. I mean I could, but I couldn't do it all together. I could only do one thing at a time. I was absolutely baffled.

It took me six years to complete a four-year kinesiology undergraduate degree, and by the fall of 1989, I had reached a crisis point because my life hadn't started. It completely fell apart. I went into a severe depression, to the point where I was sleeping for substantial amounts of time each day. I would work, barely get through the day, and then come home and sleep and sleep and sleep some more.

Added to this, I was in a five-car accident, as the one in the middle, on one of the bridges in Vancouver. This was the pièce de résistance, the icing on the cake of my life's misery. It was as though I had attracted this event in order to make sure that my external circumstances matched what I was feeling internally. No matter what I did, I felt I was the dirtiest dog, the blackest of the black. I felt there was no hope for me. In this place of darkness, I seriously considered ending it all. I just couldn't grasp how others could want to live. I couldn't reconcile how I was feeling, the heaviness, the darkness, the futility of it all. I kept repeating a damned-if-I-do-damned-if-I-don't pattern in my relationships. My only escape from these thoughts and feelings, albeit only temporary, was to numb the pain through practising a variety of addictions.

Down the Rabbit Hole

This was the darkness of my first personal bottom. I just couldn't escape the prison of how I thought and what I felt. I started sensing the magnitude of my own internal brokenness. I knew that what I'd been doing and how I'd been living was no longer working. That was a stark and bitter realization. Spending my life focused on some future accomplishment and/or regretting or hating the past had all my scorecards reading zero. I had spent the first twenty-four years of my life medicating the pain, while flipping back and forth from the past to the future. It's said that the definition of insanity is doing the same thing over and over, expecting different results. I had to admit that what I had been doing for as long as I could remember easily fit that definition.

Ignorance no longer worked and I had no idea how far I was down the rabbit hole of denial. Denial truly was one of my greatest coping mechanisms. It allowed me to convince myself that black was white, up was down, and left was right regarding the reality of my life. I was rigid, approaching life with a fear-based perfectionism that created anxiety and emotional instability. I had a continual fear of disapproval or disappointment, fear of failure or success, fear of shame, and last but not least, fear of punishment or annihilation. I was at the end of my rope and in full flight from reality. I had reached the end of the line. I could no longer kick the can of denial down the road anymore.

All I knew for sure was that I was the product of a dysfunctional alcoholic home.

Looking for Something, Anything

It was at this point that I started looking for something, anything that could give me answers. The little bit of knowledge I had about God came from my maternal grandmother. Her God was one of harshness and retribution. That old Lutheran perspective was all I had and it didn't help with how I felt at the time. I started reading the Bible. That didn't help much either, because the Old Testament just seemed to support Grandma's perspective.

I eventually found a show on television entitled T*he World Tomorrow* , hosted by Garner Ted Armstrong. I found that I was able to feel a little stillness when I watched that program. I even started to pray although I had no idea what I was doing.

During this time my mother called and told me that she had been contacted by Wendy, the wife of my biological father. Wendy was in town upgrading her medical training and she wanted to contact me. I was given Wendy's number and the choice to reach out to her or not. Eventually I did, because I figured things couldn't get much worse.

To my surprise I noticed that each time I talked with Wendy, I experienced a feeling of peace that I had never really felt before. Our interactions increased and she invited me to her apartment for supper. She was kind and aware of the animosity held toward her husband by my mother. Over time, I felt safe and open with Wendy. I started to ask her questions about faith, spirituality, and religion.

I started with the three basic questions I had always had.

Who am I?

Where did I come from?

Where can I go?

No one had ever answered them in a way that made sense

or felt right. Eventually, Wendy introduced me to some young missionaries from her church, the Church of Jesus Christ of Latter-Day Saints. Little did I know then how much my life was about to change.

My Heart Is Filled with Hope

When the missionaries explained God's Plan to me they answered my three basic questions. The information felt true and filled me with hope. It made sense. It nurtured me and it resonated deep within my heart. For the first time in my life, I felt that I was worth something. I remember the feeling of awe when I realized that in order for me to be here, on the earth, in a mortal body, I had followed Jesus Christ in the pre-mortal world. I am a child of God and I chose to stand up to defend something that is good, right, and true. This was the turning point in my life and the catalyst for change.

At the age of twenty-five, I chose to join the Church of Jesus Christ of Latter-Day Saints and was baptized on October 13, 1990. The testimony I had received at that point became the new foundation and footings in my life. It became the space and place from which I began taking my first tentative steps toward genuine healing and recovery.

Within two years I was newly married and back in school studying to be a massage therapist. This was good, but once I was in practice I started to waver in my healing journey. I had been riding the wave of my conversion and filling my life with good acts of Christian service. This isn't a bad thing, but I was doing it for the wrong reasons. Being busy serving others helped me avoid feeling my emotions. I saw that my old thought patterns and addictions were alive and well, just beneath the surface. Every time I allowed myself to be still, feelings of being unworthy and worthless were right there again, staring me in the face.

Life tends to have a way of drawing us back to those things that aren't right or resolved, and despite my best efforts to control my addictions, I started backsliding and going through the control-release cycle more and more frequently. The core feelings of shame were simply too much to bear.

I was pretty much a basket case when our first daughter was born in 1997. The prospect of being a father simply terrified me. I just consciously didn't know or understand why. The second birthday of my daughter in 1999 triggered my first sexual abuse memory.

That was a scary time for me and I consider it to be my second personal bottom, perfectly orchestrated and divinely timed by God. I distinctly remember the night I knelt in desperate heartfelt prayer and covenanted with God that I was willing to do anything and everything to break the chains of addiction and sexual abuse. This was another very real and intense choice point in my life. On some level I knew that I had reached the end of the line again, and the stakes were higher now because there was an innocent child in my home who looked to me for love and nurturance. How could I give her something that I had never received myself? I had no clue how to do this, and it filled me with an overwhelming sense of inadequacy.

12 Step Programs

Within two weeks of that prayer, I was in my first session with the alcohol and drug counsellor who has been my talk therapist ever since. Addiction recovery is really a simple two-pronged approach. First, deal with the underlying causes and conditions and second, reduce, eliminate, and replace the negative habitual patterns.

I was strongly encouraged to start attending various 12 Step programs. For me, working with a talk therapist with personal 12 Step experience has been invaluable. Gaining personal experience by repeatedly working through the 12 Steps in a group format has been critical. Together these have helped me peel back the layers of denial and reveal the underlying causes and conditions of my struggles. Working through the 12 Steps is simple but not always easy. They have brought me face to face with the truths that I had been numbing and running from throughout my life. I've found the courage to undertake new actions and face the fear of the unknown by working the 12 Steps. It's where I found the willingness to turn the flashlight back on myself, to look inward, and honestly take stock. For me there is a direct linear relationship—the more you put into working the 12 Steps, the more you'll receive from them.

All 12 Step programs are inclusive and spiritual in nature. They encourage participants to draw near and develop a personal relationship with their Higher Power. Step 12 talks about having a spiritual awakening as a result of working the eleven preceding steps. For me, personally working and repeating the 12 Steps has created repeated spiritual awakenings, every time. A spiritual awakening isn't always easy to define, but I feel that something inside of me changes. Sometimes, the spiritual awakenings are lovely pink-cloud moments and other times they're not. It retrospect, each spiritual awakening is exactly what I've needed in the moment to move forward in my recovery. They slowly help me give away everything that separates me from God, me from others, and me from myself.

Each Anonymous Program I've attended has given me new tools and skills for living. I've found many priceless gifts through reading and absorbing the literature, and associating with others who've walked through similar life experiences. This is one of the places where I fully embrace the power of association. I know that most attending the meeting will understand aspects of what I'm going through. That feeling of being accepted and understood has been, and continues to be, a key element in my personal healing. My concept of God continues to evolve and grow as I'm influenced through the love and example of others.

In my opinion, the longer I've been in recovery, the more and more honest I've become with myself. Honesty comes gradually and really becomes the flashlight that allows me to see myself as I truly am, with my strengths, weaknesses, and infirmities. Honesty allows me to bring my personal foibles and frailties into the light. As I do so, I am humbled to realize that by myself I can't change them. I don't possess the power to change them, but my Higher Power, the God of my understanding is the one Source with the power to heal my foibles and frailties.

It's clear to me that accepting my powerlessness is coupled with a willingness to trust God. Willingness is like honesty, I can never have too much of it. In my experience, there have been plenty of times when I've been resistant and unwilling to look at something in myself, often due to fear. At those times all I can do is pray—pray for the willingness to trust. If that doesn't work then I pray for the willingness to become willing. If that doesn't work then I pray for the willingness to become willing to become willing. You get the point. I will back up to where I find my faith and then I start taking my baby steps forward from there.

Re-Parenting My Inner Child

In my childhood, I had a mom and a dad in name; I called them that. But I really didn't want to believe or know that the people I called "Mom" and "Dad" knowingly, willingly, and repeatedly did terrible things or allowed others to do terrible things to me. Negative and abusive actions and behaviours that impacted me emotionally, spiritually, and psychologically, and were harmful to my physical body are simply not the actions of a mom or a dad. They are clearly the actions of individuals who lack basic human kindness and respect for other human beings. They are actions of individuals who view children as commodities to be used and sold.

It took me a long time to face any of that. My veneer was very thick and it took time to get down to the truth.

Now I realize that no one is perfect; there is no such thing as perfection. Everyone else at some point falls short. That's normal. But there is a difference between falling short out of ignorance (making genuine human mistakes) and falling short with knowledge and malicious intent.

Continually accepting my powerlessness has been an integral part of my recovery. I was ripped off from having a childhood. I was ripped off from childhood's innocence. I was ripped off from being loved unconditionally. And I can't go back and change any of it. Going back inside and dealing with memories of abuse and trauma isn't enjoyable. The process has ebbed and flowed, and I have had to face and feel some rather horrific things. In my experience, it's these horrific things that are the underlying root causes and conditions of my pain. I know that I can't do this kind of healing work by myself. I need to have help pulling out the thorns in order for my wounds to heal.

Acceptance allows me the time and patience to re-parent my inner child and be the mom and dad I never had. It takes effort, time, money, and often bloody hard work. In recovery there is a slogan; "one day at a time." Well, sometimes it comes down to a minute at a time, when things have been really tough or it's been really hard to feel my emotions and stay with them. Taking it a minute at a time, trusting my Higher Power, and remembering to breathe can get me through the next minute, the next five minutes, or however many minutes or hours are still left in the day. Things are not always at that depth of intensity, but because the truth of my childhood is brutal and hard, I grieve. The best thing about going through the grieving cycle though is that it ends with acceptance.

An Exponential Upgrade

I'm grateful to have come out of denial and realize that I'm a survivor. I realize that I have tremendous capacity and tenacity to have functioned when there was a void of love. I did what I had to do to survive. Unwinding and letting go of those survival skills and coping mechanisms, the thought patterns, the addictions, and faulty perceptions are what recovery is about. It's like getting new eyes to see, new ears to hear, and a new heart to feel.

As a child I couldn't say or do anything against the adults so I turned everything inward and I became a master at beating myself emotionally. The emotional beating stick would come out for days and weeks and months. I came from a place of harshness and that created internal harshness. Learning to be gentle with myself is really what my whole recovery journey has been about.

Courage is not the absence of fear. It's the process of feeling the fear and doing the next right thing that's placed in front of you in the present moment. Life is just a bunch of present moments that are strung together. Discerning the next right thing and taking inspired action comprise a new way of life for me that can always be refined. I'll never get it perfect and often the uninspired choices and actions are just as instructive as the inspired ones. All choices have consequences. Healing never occurs in a vacuum and it spills over into all areas of life. I will never "arrive," but I do continue to experience increasing periods of peace and balance in my life. This alone in itself indicates that my life trajectory has been exponentially upgraded.

Offering My Life Lessons through Service

As a boy I was always looking for something outside of me to change my life. This is where I started. I simply had the desire that something could be different and that something could change. Once I got a degree my life did change, but it was an inside job. The path inward is where I found my solution, and it continues to point me upward to the God of my understanding.

It's as though all the abuse and trauma I experienced in my childhood had been used to prepare my heart to receive the answers to my three basic questions—God's Plan. I experimented and planted those truths in my heart. They became my foundation to build upon and move forward from. All that I've received since then—the emotional healing, the spiritual growth, and the nurturance—has become delicious to me. Once you step into the light, it's hard to go backwards into the dark.

The physical, mental, emotional, energetic, and spiritual components of my being are intimately interwoven. They reflect and affect each other. I choose to open up, trust, and allow life's lessons to pass through me. Nothing changes unless I choose to open up, surrender, and align my will to the will of God. That's the secret and how I accept life on life's terms. All that's really mine to give is my heart and how I spend my time. How and where I spend my time is a barometer of what I value most in life. Everything else is really just on loan and provided for me to have this mortal experience.

I experienced an increasing awareness of the limitations and ineffectiveness of the physical body approach to healing. I wondered why some clients healed quickly while others languished with chronic pain. Often, it seemed that what I did had little or no lasting effect.

At some point I came across the quote, "The doctor of the future will give no medicine, but will instruct his patient in the care of the human frame, in diet and in the cause and prevention of disease." This quote, from Thomas A Edison, was a nudge and a wake-up call to me from my Higher Power. I was personally living the truth that the physical, mental, emotional, energetic, and spiritual components of an individual are intimately interwoven. I wanted to use my awareness of that truth to facilitate healing for others.

My inability to help clients with certain conditions was due to my limited perspective as a physical practitioner. I believe that healing is an art that encompasses science, and the future of wellness lies in mind-body medicine. I moved toward modalities and techniques that approach healing from a holistic perspective. I completed two trainings with the Healers Library, both of which use muscle testing to find and release imbalances in the body. Imbalances are the early forerunners of actual physiological and structural changes not yet rooted or anchored in the physical body. There are a lot of shades of grey between black and white; similarly there are a lot of steps between healthy and unhealthy for any tissue, system, and process within the body. Identifying and releasing imbalances allows our own inherent healing power to restore homeostasis or balance to the whole person.

Living in the Present

Living in the present is a gift. Presents and gifts. The gift of presence is the greatest gift and being present in the present moment is the best way to live life. Life, which can be easily missed, is just a bunch of present moments strung together. It simply comes down to listening to the still small voice of the Spirit to discern the next right thing. Once you discern the next right thing, then you choose to undertake the inspired action or not. The choice is simple and the consequences are great.

Changing the trajectory of your life is absolutely possible if you are capable of being honest with yourself. It doesn't matter how old you are or how far down you think you have gone. There is always hope. You can always find the light if you choose to look for it. Course corrections don't have to be pretty and they don't have to be fast. Course corrections do require courage and the ability to choose faith over fear. You simply start where you are.

Practise tried and true simple things:

Pray.

Meditate.

Listen to uplifting music.

Read scripture or other inspiring texts.

Take a walk in the woods or by the sea.

Find a group or organization to join.

Talk to others and simply reach out.

What you do and how it works will be unique for you. It's never too late to take inspired actions and move toward the God of your understanding.

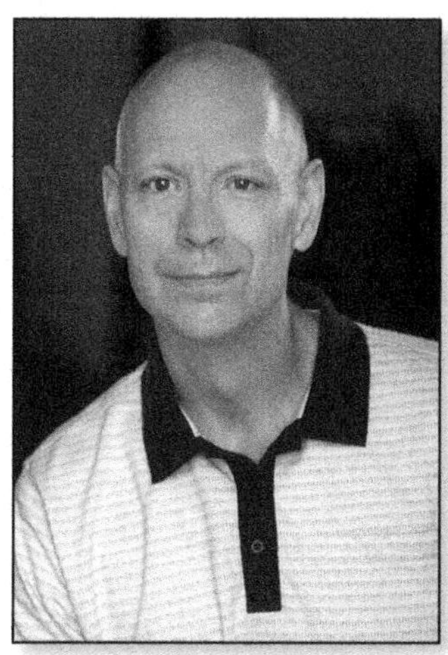

Author Biography for Kent Smith, BSc, Kinesiology; Registered Massage Therapist; Healers Library Certified Emotion Code™ Practitioner; Healers Library Certified Body Code™ Practitioner; Intuitive Healer and Coach through Heart Led Living

Kent Smith has been in practice as a Registered Massage Therapist since 1994 when he completed a 2,500-hour technical training certification at the West Coast College of Massage Therapy in New Westminster, British Columbia (BC). Prior to that, he had completed a Bachelor of Science Degree in Kinesiology at BC's Simon Fraser University in 1989.

Fifteen-plus years into his career in rehabilitation and sports-focused environments, Kent realized that the physical approach to healing was only part of the answer. He went back to school and trained with the Healers Library as a Certified Emotion Code™ Practitioner in 2010 and as a Certified Body Code™ Practitioner in 2015.

He also completed the inaugural Intuitive Healer and Coach training through Heart Led Living in 2015 and is now in the advanced mentoring program. This training has expanded Kent's perspective even more regarding the art of energy-based healing.

Kent lives in Vancouver, BC with his spouse and two daughters. He is an avid family history buff and enjoys helping others with their genealogical research. He also enjoys swimming, woodworking, and the occasional all-terrain-vehicle and snowmobile adventure.

You can reach Kent and learn more about his offerings at heartledliving.com/our-coaches/Kent-Smith/.

Chapter 4

Ready to Feel

by Diana Calvo

Ready to Feel

by Diana Calvo

I Asked God for Help

I recently began to experience miracles in my life. At an extremely low point in my life, I asked God for help, and everything began to change. After trying to pull myself out of depression for three years, it became clear that what I was doing wasn't working, and I needed help. I surrendered to a power greater than myself, I asked for help, and I received it. Over a period of six months, I have been blessed with people, messages, awarenesses, and events at the perfect times for my deepest healing to occur. I have healed childhood trauma that has been with me for forty years. I have gone from being numb to feeling. I have experienced the incredible freedom of giving myself love by honouring the true desires of my heart.

I have taken responsibility for the role I have played in my life and, in particular, the role I played in situations where I previously believed other people had wronged me. Every day I am further convinced of my worthiness, my connection to others, and my ability to access the unlimited source of love I have inside myself. I am committed to letting my heart lead me. Every time I follow my heart and choose love over fear, I am reminded how beautiful it is to be alive.

Opting Out of Feelings

As human beings, our natural state is one of equilibrium, feeling peace and love within, and experiencing good mental and physical health. Feelings are part of being human, and expressing feelings is essential to the human experience. Feelings are also energy, and the expression of feelings allows that energy to be released from our bodies so that we can return to equilibrium. Children can be excellent teachers of the way we were naturally designed to feel our feelings. We see this when a child spontaneously runs up to someone for a hug, or suddenly her eyes fill with tears and her lips begin to quiver, or his eyes and smile are shining so brightly you can see the light and feel the warmth of his heart. Regardless of the feeling, many children express themselves immediately and fully, and for as long as necessary, to allow the energy to be released from their body. Each one of us is designed to express ourselves in this way, yet life circumstances can cause us to turn away from this natural way of being. I believe the conscious choice to fully experience our feelings is absolutely necessary to be truly awake and alive during our lifetime. In other words, I believe the choice to *feel* is a choice to *live*.

For many of us, somewhere along the way, we make a

choice to stop feeling our feelings. In many cases, the choice is not a conscious one. But once the choice is made, we no longer allow the natural flow of energy in our bodies through the full expression of our emotions. When the energy isn't released, it becomes trapped in the body, creating a disequilibrium that manifests in any number of ways. For example, trapped energy can express itself as a physical symptom (a headache, a rash, an infection, a muscle ache), a mental health issue (depression, anxiety, neurosis), or the perceived inability to change unwanted life circumstances (relationships, career, home, family).

I stopped feeling my feelings shortly after I was born. I've lived my entire life with a deep sense of emptiness inside, and it is only recently that I am remembering what it is to feel solid and whole and alive. Fear was one reason I opted out of feeling my feelings.

For one thing, I was born into my family's story that says it isn't safe to be who you are. I have German heritage on one side and, even though my grandfather was a United States soldier in World War II, my grandparents did not feel safe in openly sharing our German ancestry.

On the other side of my family there is Jewish heritage, something my parents kept a very closely guarded secret. I imagine my family was genuinely afraid of prejudices and hatred that felt very real and dangerous to them at the time. As a child, I could sense these fearful feelings in the adults around me. However, we didn't talk about these things very much, and a fear of exposing who I really am remained unaddressed in my subconscious belief system for many years.

Another reason I stopped feeling my feelings was my fear of experiencing the painful emotions associated with my childhood. I am the adult child of a narcissistic mother. Narcissism is a personality disorder recognized by the *Diagnostic and Statistical*

Manual of Mental Disorders (DSM–5). Because of my mother's narcissism, I experienced emotional abuse as a child and this negatively impacted my own emotional development. One example of the effect my mother's narcissism had on me is that, as a child, I believed that my existence was problematic for everyone. In particular, I believed that I was a serious burden on my mother. On more than one occasion, she let me know in no uncertain terms that, given everything on her plate, she didn't have the resources—time, money, attention, love—to take care of me. This is an emotionally devastating message for a child and it was more than I could handle. Not feeling so as to avoid this pain was a coping mechanism that was necessary for my growth and survival.

Also in response to believing I was a burden, I tried to make myself disappear. Outwardly, I always did what I was told so that no one got upset with me. I spoke very little, I never expressed a contrary opinion, and I spent a lot of time alone. Inwardly, I was obsessively concerned with the emotions of the adults around me (especially those of my mother), and I went to great lengths to try and make sure everyone was always feeling okay. This behaviour continued well into my adult years. In retrospect, I see that I experienced a very unhealthy loss of my own sense of self as I focused all my attention on the emotional needs of others. My fear of feeling the emotional pain from my childhood kept me continually looking outside myself. Because I dared not look inward where the pain was, I never really got to know myself. Not having answers to questions about my true interests, desires, gifts, likes, dislikes, and passions contributed to my growing sense of emptiness.

I experienced emptiness as a vague, but always present, physical discomfort throughout my entire body. I also had a sense of uneasiness in everything I experienced, and a deep knowing that something unidentifiable about my life was fundamentally wrong. I always sensed my own darkness, but it had been there so consistently and for so long that I couldn't remember anything else. The darkness was hidden in plain sight, just the way things were. This was a far cry from living in peace, love, and equilibrium, to which the body is always trying to return. Returning to such a state would require me to face my fears, experience the emotional pain I had been avoiding my whole life and, in so doing, allow the energy of those emotions to be released from my body.

At the age of thirty-three, I made the decision to no longer communicate with anyone in my family. This was after a difficult visit with my mother and brother. Visits always triggered the potential release of painful emotions that I wasn't ready to feel.

By now the physical and emotional discomfort of those unexpressed emotions—the trapped energy—was growing in intensity. I needed more serious distractions to continue avoiding those feelings. I began to overeat and I developed an addiction to food. Every time my true painful feelings of grief, anger, rage, and sadness threatened to express themselves, I would eat something to avoid them. I also ate to try and bury the growing sensation of emptiness I was experiencing. My life revolved around what to eat next. Meals and snacks were what I looked forward to throughout the day, every day. I ate until I was uncomfortably full and then I kept eating. I had developed regular afternoon headaches that I remedied with twice-daily doses of over-the-counter painkillers. My digestive tract was seriously inflamed and I was diagnosed with a stomach ulcer. I was constantly dealing with the entire gamut of digestive issues.

I remember the day I realized that my eating was out of control. Coming off a period of binge eating during the holidays, my body was screaming for me to stop. I was experiencing a lot of physical pain. I could clearly see the linkage between my overeating and the physical pain in my body, and yet I couldn't stop putting food in my mouth. It was a very humbling and scary time in my life. I admitted to myself I didn't know how to fix things and I needed help.

I came across "The Clean Program," a philosophy around food and eating in modern times. The program includes a twenty-one-day cleanse and lifetime phone support. I signed up. It was this program that introduced me to the idea of eating to avoid feeling our feelings. I came to realize that was exactly what I was doing. Becoming conscious of the connection between overeating and avoiding feelings in my life was an important step in my journey of spiritual awakening. The conscious awareness also freed me, over time, to make different choices around food that I felt much better about, both physically and emotionally.

While I had woken up to using food to numb myself, it would still take several more years before I had the courage to fully feel the emotional pain from my childhood and to release that energy from my body.

Prayer to Feel Your Feelings

Here is a prayer I wrote to help me feel my feelings.

Dear God,

There is pain inside me, and I am afraid that feeling it is more than I can possibly handle.

I fear the pain is so great that I will literally die if I allow myself to feel it.

I realize that I have spent a lifetime trying to protect myself from this pain, and I don't blame myself for that. I had my reasons for doing so.

I am now beginning to understand that I am a prisoner to this pain trapped in my body.

I long for freedom from this suffering.

I don't know what to do.

I am asking for your help.

Please show me the way, one step at a time, to be able to face my fears and feel my feelings, no matter how painful they may be.

Please help me to remember my own strength and courage, so that I may set myself free.

Amen

Returning to Feelings

If we have been emotionally numb for most of our lives, we need to re-learn how to feel our feelings. The numbness is the result of subconsciously deciding, over and over again, to avoid feelings and to not allow the energy of our emotions to be released from our bodies. Over time this numbness can become the routine way in which we experience the world. Without expressing our emotions, we live in our minds as opposed to our hearts. We can't live fully when we live in the mind. Living in the mind creates a feeling of disconnection from ourselves and from others. In addition, we can't live in the mind and simultaneously acknowledge all of the different components of our being—mind, heart, body, soul—which can leave us feeling incomplete or internally at odds with ourselves.

When re-learning how to feel, it is so important to remember that feelings are energy in the body. Feelings are not the same as thoughts and we need to make the distinction between the two. We can't look for feelings in our minds, we have to look in our bodies. There are three parts to this process of re-learning. The first part is the conscious awareness of our own numbness and the desire to no longer be numb. The second part is developing the ability to look inward and become consciously aware of what is happening within the body. The third part is sitting with what is happening inside the body and observing it with patience and curiosity.

I met my ex-husband when I was twenty-eight and we married when I was thirty. We divorced eight years later. While I was married, and even through my divorce, I could sense, but still could not articulate, the feelings of emptiness inside me. I was still emotionally numb and lacking self-love and self-esteem. Subconsciously, while I was married, I looked to my husband to fix my feelings of emptiness, and to make me feel that everything was okay. While there were many factors that contributed to our divorce, I take responsibility for the part I played in the difficulties of our marriage. The expectations I placed on my husband to meet my emotional needs were unreasonable. I have since come to understand that true and lasting feelings of wholeness, peace, and love are feelings that come from deep within ourselves. I had mistakenly been looking for them in another person.

One of the biggest challenges I have faced as I re-learn how to feel is that I need to surrender and to allow good things to happen naturally. I need to let go of trying to control everything that happens in my life. Trying to control creates an illusion of safety that I want so badly to believe is real. I need to trust that my life is worth something in and of itself, and that I'm taken care of by a power much larger than myself. I need to allow that larger power to work through me, to guide me, to show me whatever it is I'm meant to see. My trust grows every time I allow myself to feel. I am still grieving my relationship with my family, my childhood circumstances, and the years I've been asleep in my life. I want to be done grieving and I want to be feeling great all the time. So I keep choosing, over and over again, to surrender to what is actually happening in my body, good or bad, and to express the feelings. Every time I allow myself to feel the feelings fully, I experience relief as the energy moves through my body. And slowly I come to understand the bad feelings are not the whole truth of who I am.

My Experience with Depression

It was my experience with depression that led me to make a commitment to feeling my feelings fully in my own life. Depression for me looked like a severe lack of energy, disinterest in life, social withdrawal, and a vague sense of pointlessness and dread hovering over me wherever I went. My depression grew slowly but steadily over a period of three years. I woke up to the seriousness of it one day when, after a breakfast meeting for work, I was so exhausted that I had to cancel the rest of my commitments for the day and go home to bed. Sleeping in the middle of the day in the middle of the work week was such a strange occurrence for me that it woke me up to the fact that something was seriously wrong in my life.

At the age of forty-one, I looked at my life and didn't like what I saw. My lifelong dream of living in a beautiful home was still not realized, despite owning a home and having spent twenty years successfully climbing the corporate ladder. At the height of my career, I had lost interest in my work and was just going through the motions. I had started up again with poor eating habits and not exercising, even though I knew better. I had fallen into a depression and not even realized it. I didn't know who I was or what I wanted. I was asleep in my life.

During the same three-year period, while experiencing a

growing sense of dissatisfaction with my job, I began to explore alternative career options, asking myself what kind of work might make me happy. No matter how much I thought about it, my question was answered with my own silence and blank stare. I was frustrated and at a complete loss for what to do, and so I met with a career coach. After reading the answers I provided to her list of detailed questions, and talking with me on the phone, she concluded that my issues at work had nothing to do with my work and everything to do with the fact that I was the adult child of a narcissistic mother. She provided me with some resources on narcissism, suggested I do my own research, and let me know there was nothing for us to do around work until these deeper issues were resolved.

As part of my research on narcissism, I learned the important role grieving has for a successful recovery. I needed to grieve for the years I spent numb and not living fully. I needed to grieve for the fact that I missed out on experiencing a mother's unconditional love, and that as an adult I no longer had any right to expect that from anyone other than myself. I needed to grieve for the suffering I experienced as a little girl in an extremely unfortunate situation. I needed to grieve for the anger and rage I felt toward my mother for the things she did. I knew that I had buried my grief deep inside me. I believe that experiencing the grief was essential for my healing. I also knew I had buried unexpressed feelings of sadness, anger, rage, resentment, and guilt. These feelings—and their associated energies—had been unexpressed and trapped in my body for years. The depression was my final wake-up call that I couldn't continue to live this way.

When I decided to pull myself out of depression, I started looking at my life honestly. Through my own introspection, supported by healers, I began to realize that all my suffering ultimately came back around to the emotional pain I was avoiding. Those trapped emotions were running the show by subconsciously influencing my thoughts, feelings, and behaviours. In order to avoid feeling, I was making choices that were keeping me stuck in circumstances I didn't really want. Avoiding these feelings was costing me a lot. It was costing me my life. Not changing was more terrifying than changing.

I was ready to wake up and start living. My choice to live was a choice to feel. Earlier in my life I had made the connection between my addictive behaviours as a way to avoid feeling. I was now ready to start feeling.

I put myself on a healing regime of weekly yoga, therapy, and energy healing with the hopes that I could discover how to feel my grief with the help of these healers. Each one played an important role for which I will be forever grateful. But it was the energy healer who had the most profound impact on my life. With her assistance, I was able to make the connection between my body and my emotions, and I began to experience for myself the sensation of an emotion trapped in my body, and then its release. I began to re-learn how to feel my feelings, and the grieving process began.

Exercise to Feel Your Feelings

This is an exercise I developed to release trapped emotions from my body.

1. When you notice an unpleasant physical sensation in your body, immediately stop what you are doing and find a place where you can be alone and free of distraction.
2. Sit down or lie down, whichever you prefer.
3. Close your eyes. Be still. Be quiet.
4. Focus your attention fully on the unpleasant physical

sensation. Look at it directly. Notice everything about it that you can.

   a. Where is the feeling located in your body? For example, is it in your chest, diaphragm, forehead?
   b. What does it feel like? For example, is it pressing, squeezing, pinching.
   c. How is it moving? For example, is it pushing outwards from the inside, rising upwards, zipping around in circles?
   d. Is there something you can compare it to? For example, is it like nausea, a steel rod, a rope, a breeze?

5. Stay focused on the physical sensation and continue to observe it with patience and curiosity.
6. If you notice the physical sensation turning into an emotion, welcome the emotion, and allow it to be expressed as fully as you can, and for as long as you are able.
7. When the experience is complete, acknowledge and appreciate yourself for choosing to face the unpleasant physical sensation, and for choosing to allow the experience that occurred, whatever it was.
8. Reflect on your experience and consider writing about it in a personal journal. Writing can be a wonderful way to further connect with your experience and to acknowledge your progress over time.
9. Celebrate yourself for honouring your desire to live fully through this experience.

Freedom in Feeling

When we make the conscious decision to feel our feelings fully, we can experience the freedom that comes from finally letting those feelings go. It's a decision that requires a real commitment. The commitment is to look directly and honestly at our life, our family, our experiences, our relationships, and our role in the whole thing. Then, we need to feel all the accompanying feelings that go with it, no matter how painful those feelings may be, no matter how terrified we are, no matter how long it takes, and no matter how tired we are of rehashing the same old stories.

An important part of feeling my feelings was starting to reconnect with my heart and the feeling of love. I could sense that I had some very thick walls constructed around my heart. I also felt that my heart was frozen. I was attending an event for women entrepreneurs when one of the women shared some of her life story. She had suffered trauma as a child and now, as an adult, she had developed an allergy to sunlight. Her skin would break out in a rash if she was exposed to direct sunlight. As you can imagine this was significantly restricting her life experiences. As she told her story, I could feel her emotional suffering related to her allergy, and I could feel her fear and avoidance of the pain of her childhood trauma. I saw a lot of similarities between her story and my own. I can remember the feeling of love I had for her in that moment as she shared her story. I literally felt my heart crack open—just a teeny tiny bit—and could sense my love for her pouring out of my chest in a ray of light. The strength of the love energy, combined with my lack of practice around feeling love, left me with a sensitive bruising sensation in my chest. The feeling of my heart cracking is what clued me in to my frozen heart that was now beginning to thaw.

In addition to giving love to others, I also started to experiment with giving love to myself. I discovered that a sense of obligation to others, and to meeting their needs, was subconsciously dictating some of my behaviour. I was doing things I didn't truly want to do in order to please other people, and then feeling that uncomfortable gnawing away inside because I wasn't being true to myself.

Saying no to other people is one of the ways I sometimes give love to myself. For example, I hired an interior designer to help me decorate my home. When the project was finished, she was interested in photographing the apartment to showcase it on her website in support of further developing her interior design business. She had photographed it once before, and so this would be the second photoshoot. When she made the request, I could feel a squeezing sensation throughout my entire torso, and I knew my body was telling me something about the true feelings in my heart. When I stopped to listen, I realized that I was going through a period when a lot of grief was rising up and out at unexpected times. I needed the security of knowing I had a private space where I could cry whenever I needed to. I couldn't commit to a photoshoot and feel good about it. I made the choice to show myself love by honouring my true feelings and desires.

When I responded to the interior designer, I didn't make excuses. I was honest with her and let her know that as much as I wanted to support her in growing her business, I was going through some personal things and couldn't commit to the photoshoot at the moment. For me, this was an incredibly new, liberating, and joyful way to be in the world. I first connected with my true feelings about a situation and then I made sure my actions and my words were in alignment with those feelings.

While I am no longer in a state of depression, I still have days when unhelpful thoughts enter my mind and I experience dark feelings. Sometimes I will have thoughts that my life is pointless and it doesn't matter. When those thoughts come,

I feel alone and disconnected. I don't feel a yes for life in my heart. I can become overwhelmed, sensing a lack of purpose and no reason for being. I've learned that when this darkness visits me, avoiding and ignoring the feelings only prolongs my suffering. On the other hand, when I accept the feelings as what I am experiencing in the moment, and I allow the feelings to be expressed fully, the dark energy is released and I return to equilibrium. I can once again feel peace and love in my heart. I return to a place of hope.

Where I have struggled the most to feel my feelings is in connection with receiving love from others. Based on my relationship with my family during my childhood, I developed the unconscious belief that receiving love is associated with pain and danger. This belief has kept me closed off from receiving love from other people, which is a fundamental part of being human and being alive. I feel a deep sadness when I reflect on how I have kept other people at a distance for so much of my life. It's humbling to realize the role I played in my own feelings of loneliness and isolation.

I'm grateful that I'm choosing differently now. I make a conscious effort in my day-to-day life to be open to receiving love. Here are some of the ways I allow myself to feel love from others:

- joyfully accepting and embracing offers of help
- receiving compliments without interrupting
- responding to compliments with a genuine thank you
- sharing myself with others
- welcoming the attention of others
- giving and receiving real hugs

Mantra to Feel My Feelings

Here is a mantra I use to feel my feelings.

I choose to feel my feelings fully.

I choose to release energy that is trapped in my body.

I choose to surrender completely to any painful emotions associated with past experiences.

I choose to welcome new feelings in each moment of every day.

I choose to love all my feelings, including those I judge to be good and those I judge to be bad.

I choose to recognize myself as separate from my feelings, and to let each feeling gently come and gently go.

Returning to Love

The first forty years of my life consisted of a lot of leaving. I left my father when I was fifteen. I left my brother when I was eighteen. I left my mother when I was thirty-three. I left my husband when I was thirty-eight. I left my career when I was forty. All of this leaving was an outward expression of my inner reality, where I had been leaving my own self. I abandoned myself every time I decided to avoid my own feelings, ignore the truth of my own experiences, and focus all my interest on the needs of others without putting any time or effort into getting to know myself.

After I left my job, from an external point of view, there was nothing left to leave. The only leaving that remained was to leave my life. It was at that point, in the darkest and scariest times of my depression, that my heart made itself known. I followed the guidance of my heart and started myself on a path of healing. I made the decision to never abandon myself again.

That meant staying. That meant looking at my life with honesty and eyes wide open. That meant feeling everything that needed to be felt, from the past and the present.

Since leaving my job, I find myself doing the most important work of my life. I am dedicating this year to getting to know myself and what my purpose is during this lifetime. Right now, I am letting go of things on an epic scale. I am letting go of my own pain and fear. I am letting go of what everyone else thinks, wants, and expects. I am letting go of my attachment to people and outcomes. I am letting go of wanting to be in control. I am letting go of choosing from among the options presented by the status quo.

Through this process of emptying, I am making room for new things to come into my life. I know I am on the right track because I feel more alive now than ever before. I am no longer abandoning myself! This fills me with so much self-love and self-esteem. I see all of my life—even the pain and the challenges—as purposeful in leading me to exactly this time and place of rebirth and renewal. I am immensely grateful for all my years of working in a job and my savings from that work, which are allowing me this time to travel inward, to heal, and in a wonderful way, to begin again.

Since I started this healing journey, I have experienced the feeling of joy for the first time in my life. I have had moments of feeling the oneness of everything, my connection to another, my connection to all others, the connection of all others to each other, and the connection of all of us to a universal source. I have had days when positive energy is pulsing through my body and I am full of love and hope. I also have days full of grief, and days that are full of darkness. There are times when fear is guiding me, and times when love is guiding me. My hope and desire are to continually live with more conscious awareness, more in the present, more allowing of everything, more attached to nothing, and more fully guided by love. I've experienced rare moments with another person, when we both speak and share our truth from our hearts. In these moments, we create a beautiful space where I feel completely free and fully alive. I wish this, and more, for the next forty years of my life, and for you.

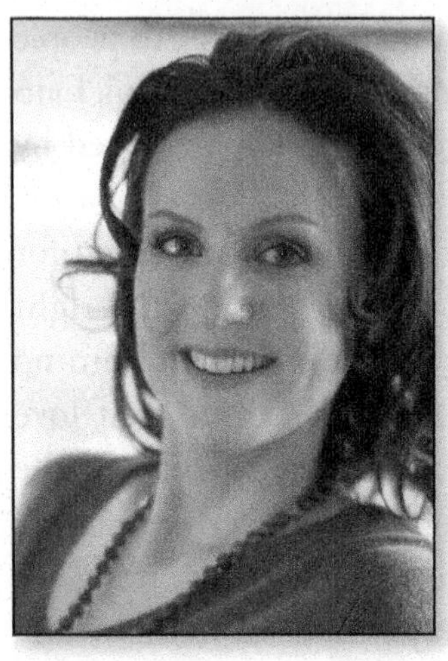

Author Biography for Diana Calvo , Former Corporate Executive, Coach and Mentor. Currently taking time off and creating a new life.

Diana Calvo lives in the United States, studied economics in college, and spent twenty years successfully climbing the corporate ladder. At the age of forty, she faced an overwhelming sense of dissatisfaction with her life and how she was living it. She took a leap, left her corporate career, and embarked on a journey of healing and self-discovery. She has personally experienced a spiritual awakening through deep exploration of her inner self. Along the way, she has practised many forms of the healing arts, including yoga, meditation, and energy healing. She is a member of Sue Dumais's Heart Led Living community and is committed to letting her heart lead.

To learn more about Diana and her offerings, visit diana-calvo.com.

Chapter 5

Releasing Anxiety, Embracing Faith

by Rachel Shoniker

Releasing Anxiety, Embracing Faith

by Rachel Shoniker

Swimming in Stress

"You're a Libra with a Gemini rising! This makes you light and playful. Oh, but wait, there is this worry that you've inherited from your mother."

My heart sank as the astrologer interpreted my chart and shared my verdict. A unanimous jury. I was to be sentenced to a life of stress, worry, and fear. (Or so it felt at the time.) I desperately wanted to be light and playful!

I used to joke that I was born stressed out. Unfortunately, this was more of a truth than a far-fetched joke. In 2006, a first-time visit to a hypnotherapist in Vancouver, Canada, changed my understanding of who I really am. With eyes closed, I watched in awe as a tiny butterfly of radiant light fluttered toward me and then determinedly dove into my fetus body. For a fleeting moment, I felt a deep sense of joy, excitement, and love. Then, without warning, this infinite joy was sucker punched by a thick, sickly feeling of worry and fear. These toxic emotions belonged to my young pregnant mom. The vibrating bundle of love and joy that I observed was (is) my true essence—my soul. Here was the light and playful part of me!

Unfortunately, for most of my life, anxiety and fear were the dangerous drivers steering my experiences, perspectives, and emotions.

Five Years Old and All Grown Up

Fragile, pale, and beautiful, my young mom sat beside me at the kitchen table. The mouthwatering smell of homemade soup wrapped the room in a familiar blanket. Surrounded in Austria by my mother's extended family, I sat quietly, observing the scene. My mom's female cousin, the chef of the house, owned the spotlight and chatted incessantly. While the atmosphere seemed lively, it wasn't powerful enough to quell the heavy emotions within me. Weighed down with the cumbersome energy of my depressed mom, I felt like an overly serious adult trapped in a five-year-old's body. Overwhelmed and alone.

After meeting my Canadian dad in a ski resort in the Austrian Alps while she was working there, my nineteen-year old mom ran away to Canada. In love and allured by the dream of a comfortable and secure family life, my mom married my dad shortly after they started dating. The initial years of family life were challenging for my twenty-something-year-old mom. Living in a foreign country—Canada—she had made few friends and had no relatives. She worried chronically that my young father wouldn't be able to provide for us. Her fear of poverty stemmed from her early childhood years. She had been raised in Austria by her grandmother, and the basic necessities of food and clothing had been a struggle to come by.

Mostly, my mom was consumed with guilt about leaving her relatives, especially her grandmother. Mom's grandmother fought hard to get my mom to return, targeting her with endless missiles of guilt. After surviving the death of two husbands and two adult children, my great-grandmother didn't want to lose my mom too.

Like a heavy, rusted chain anchoring a boat to the ocean floor, guilt kept my young mom stuck and unable to sail free. Finally, she decided to leave my dad behind in Canada and move my little brother and me to the farming village in Austria where her relatives lived.

Her mind was consumed with doubt and fear; her heart was heavy with sorrow. And little five-year old me felt it all. Energetically, I desperately tried to absorb her despair. I longed for my mom to be happy. I longed for her to unleash herself from that rusty, heavy anchor and sail free.

After my mom, my brother, and I had been away for nearly one year, my dad insisted that we return to Canada and live as a family. He had discovered the perfect community for us to plant our roots and grow—the nature-rich, laid-back mountain town of Nelson, in the interior of British Columbia. Our move was the beginning of a new chapter for our family.

Childhood—A Matter of Fear and Survival

Wearing a white dress with embroidered red flowers, I sat silently at my small desk. My shiny, dark brown hair stretched down my back in a long braid. Like a frightened deer that sensed a threat, I felt frozen in fear, struggling to breathe. Completely still, I prayed that nobody would notice me. For most kids, it was an average day at school. Children were learning, listening, yawning, daydreaming, playing, and teasing one another. But for me, a shy and sensitive seven-year old, every day at school felt like a dark tunnel filled with scary monsters. A frightening place where I felt completely alone. A matter of survival.

In my teens and twenties, I learned to hide my anxiety. My mask was a confident face that often came across as arrogant and unapproachable. My costumes were attention-grabbing ensembles. Wearing colourful, 1960s-inspired retro outfits to barely there crop tops and booty-hugging mini dresses, the character I channeled was showy and fearless. A desperate attempt to deny and ignore the way I felt inside. Inevitably, signs of my inner anxiety and feelings of unworthiness began popping up. My lack of self-love, buried fears, and denied sadness manifested into eating disorders, substance abuse, and anxiety attacks. Deep into my late thirties, an intense, knotted ball of anxiety was a permanent resident in my gut.

A Song for Healing

On a warm evening in the spring of 2005, I found myself at a book signing event. A slender woman with a crisp white blouse stood at the front of a small audience. Successful and bright, she seemed to have her life under control. She began her presentation by singing a heartfelt song about her personal journey. The author's words of struggle with anxiety and feelings of unworthiness plunged into my heart.

Like a mountain creek after a big snowmelt, endless tears streamed down my face. Embarrassed, I desperately choked back childlike sobs. Her singing had unlocked a hidden door to a dark room of sadness within me. That evening, at thirty years old, I had a startling epiphany. Not only did I not like myself, but I loathed myself. With this shocking awareness, my healing journey had officially begun.

My journey to self-love and healing would be a slow, potholed road with unplanned detours and wonderful insights. It was less like a smooth highway with oversized, easy-to-read signs and more like a twisty country road, the scenic route that kept me wondering and curious and sometimes confused and doubtful. Was there anyone out there who could help me navigate the road? I would find my sage teacher and guide, Sue Dumais, nearly a decade later.

Meditation and Clairvoyance Find Me

On a hot August day in Vancouver, my non-air-conditioned office felt claustrophobic. Desperate for air, I opened the windows wide, only to be hit with noisy traffic and zero breeze. With my breath growing increasingly shallow, I anxiously waited to escape outside to a nearby waterfront park. But it wasn't the summer heat that was the source of my stress. My anxiety had reached a staggering, all-time high. The Everest of anxiety peaks.

My boyfriend at the time (a guy with whom I had a decade-long, on-again-off-again relationship) had gotten himself into some big-time problems with the law. While I always knew that he was no model citizen, this shocking event sent me spinning like a toy top. I couldn't think. I couldn't work. I couldn't function. My anxiety was larger than me. Then, unexpectedly, on that summer day in 2008, the Universe delivered a sign, showed me the way out of my dark tunnel, and pointed me toward my destined path as a clairvoyant.

In my office sat a dark-haired forty-something-year-old man. He was a smoker who had supposedly contacted me to help him quit. Dizzy from intense anxiety, I robotically walked him through a consultation. When our meeting approached its end, he suddenly asked if I would be interested in receiving an energy healing. To which, I heard myself desperately shout: "Yes, please!"

Like an iron smoothing out a crumpled dress, a silky, flowy sensation replaced my extreme anxiety. It was as if someone had combed out the mangled mess of energy in my body and mind. The following day, I called the stranger and requested to hire him for more energy healing treatments. His response was not what I wanted to hear: "No, but you can learn to do this yourself." With that, he gave me the name of a colleague teaching an upcoming course.

Spirit was clearly pointing me in the direction that would allow me to uncover my intuitive gifts and awaken the dormant healer within me. At the time, I couldn't see the obvious sign. I wanted to be healed … and now. I wanted someone to save me. My fear-based, victimhood state of mind had me blinded. Seven months later, I was ready to follow Spirit's guidance.

In April 2009, I participated in the first of several meditation and energy healing programs. Meditation quickly became my new, trusted companion. Something I could rely on to help me feel calmer. A practice that allowed me to connect to something far greater than myself, a loving Source that was always supporting me. I was relieved to know that I wasn't alone trying to find my way through life.

The workshop also had some mystifying surprises. On the second day of class, the instructor asked me to do a reading of a woman in Iran. Having no clue how to conduct a reading, I closed my eyes and waited nervously for something to happen.

I didn't wait long. Defined, colour-rich images appeared in front of my closed eyes. Blazing red adrenal glands pumped full of anger and resentment. Black spots peppered her lungs. Years later, I discovered that this woman would be hospitalized with a serious lung infection.

A second attempt at a reading, this time with a young woman in England, revealed an intestinal tract coated with something greyish, smothering, and harmful. When I reported what I saw, a workshop participant shared that his British friend had recently attempted to end her life by drinking poison.

At the time, I couldn't understand how or why I was seeing what I was seeing. But I did know that it wasn't me who was responsible for these images and information. I was simply a channel, a messenger, a conduit.

Silent Retreat at White-Knuckle Speed

In spring 2010, I attended a ten-day silent meditation retreat. My financial and emotional wellbeing had been free falling into a bottomless, black hole for a while. I longed to feel peace. But instead of experiencing meditation bliss, the heightened vibration of being surrounded by forty-five fellow meditators intensified my clairvoyance. Non-stop images hurled themselves at me at a nauseating speed.

I was shown different realms—the quirkiness and beauty of which I could have never imagined. I witnessed emotional events from early childhood of which I had no conscious memory. With eyes resting closed, past lives unfolded like thriller movies. The betrayals and deaths felt fearfully real. Historical and spiritual images flew at me at white-knuckle speed. At one point, my friend's deceased bulldog, Hugo, even visited me with a message for her!

Finally, on day ten, the flood of information ceased, permitting me to experience the peace I was craving. My body and mind dissolved into flowing waves of energy, dancing with the energy that surrounded me, an incredible taste of Divine bliss and unconditional love.

When Anxiety Has a Mysterious Root

Sprawled out on my husband's and my comfortable bed in our downtown Vancouver condo, I listened carefully to the soothing voice on my cell phone. The female voice explained that the chronic anxiety that plagued me had an ancestral connection that dated seven generations back on my mother's side. She shared that this specific past life had ended with the ultimate betrayal—murder. I had been killed with a sharp weapon stabbed into my upper back. For many lives, I had been carrying the intense stress of this gruesome death and devastating betrayal.

With my permission, the adept healer pulled the event's root from within me. As the memory was released from my body, my arms and legs shook frantically, uncontrollably bouncing off the bed.

The calm voice on my phone that day in September 2012 belonged to Sue Dumais, an intuitive healer who facilitates remote healings from her home on a farm outside Vancouver. Since this life-changing healing session, chronic anxiety has no longer been my unwanted roommate. The constant mangled ball of anxiety in my gut is gone.

Same Stress, Different Day

As I observed my life, I noticed that certain situations were triggering feelings of fear, anxiety, unworthiness, helplessness, loneliness, and so forth. These events and relationships were present in my life for my healing. The Universe was offering me an opportunity to look at emotions I had stored within in order to release them. Spirit peppers our lives with these uncomfortable circumstances until we have the courage to face our inner fear and sadness, allowing us to heal. If, on the contrary, we continue to protect our fears and inner hurt, keeping them hoarded within, we will never be free and truly happy.

In the past six years, I have traveled frequently. On many of my flights, there was often at least one crying baby or toddler. As if there was a bright spotlight shining on the upset infant, everything else would drift into the background. I would be unable to focus on anything else. My breath would grow shallow. Like a non-swimmer thrown into deep water, panic quickly crept through me until I was completely submerged. Unable to escape, I remained in my seat in a state of panic and fear until the mother was able to calm her distressed little one.

When I first noticed this trigger and response, I decided that it must be the curse of an empath and I desperately needed to work on my ability to ground myself. But as the years passed, the situation repeatedly occurred. Although the settings and circumstances sometimes differed, the trigger and panic response within me was always the same. Same stress, different day.

One rainy winter day, I sat in our neighbourhood community centre outside my two-year-old's dance class. I watched as one mom anxiously tried to push her toddler into the class. The toddler cried hysterically, and frantically pushed her mom back, fighting to not go in. Suddenly, I noticed a familiar sensation within me. Like an enormous ocean wave, a feeling of panic crashed over me. Judgmental, angry thoughts raced through my mind. "She doesn't want to be in the class! She's scared. She doesn't want to be separated from you, her mom. Why are you trying to make her go? You're a terrible, selfish mother."

Then, amidst my tornado of emotions, I stopped and looked around at the other moms. Some faces displayed gentle caring, while some were totally neutral and unaffected. Nobody looked like I felt inside. Nobody was in a state of raw panic.

It had become obvious to me that this was not about me being an ultrasensitive empath who could feel other people's energy; nor was this about a lack of grounding. The Divine was orchestrating these events for my own healing. The time was ripe for me to look at this anxiety and fear in order to release them and heal.

Sitting with eyes gently closed, I asked Spirit to please show me my fear. What is truly bothering me when I witness a distressed small child? Instantly, a story in images unfolded behind my closed eyes. I observed a four-year-old girl with brown hair standing at a bus station in front of a wall of baggage. One bag with a bright white tag stood out. The bag belonged to the child's mother. Tuning in to the little girl's emotions, I felt deep sadness, helplessness, and loneliness. She desperately wanted her mom to stay with her. I heard the words: "Don't leave me. I'm scared. Don't leave me alone."

With these thoughts, I saw the image of a woman's body walking briskly away in her shiny black heels and calf-length, black skirt. It felt as though she had ambitious plans. And a small child didn't fit into these plans. At the time, the mother was not coming back. Heartbroken, the girl watched her go.

Although this event did not occur in my current lifetime (the child was me in another life), the emotional memory was stashed within me. The feelings that this event triggered were very real for me in this life. Often when we look directly at the root of our fears, the information that presents itself is surprising. By witnessing this emotional past-life event in meditation, I was able to permit the fear, sadness, loneliness, and helplessness to simmer to the surface and be released.

Witnessing this past-life event represented one layer of healing for me. But I was aware that Little Rachel also harboured feelings of helplessness, loneliness, and sadness. These were feelings that I had buried within me when I was a little girl. In order for me to feel safe and loved (as well as not feel panicked when a stranger's child is distressed), it was essential for me to turn my attention inward and allow these stored emotions to be expressed and released.

The path to freedom requires feeling what is within and letting it go. Yes, there might be tears. And that's perfectly okay. As my teacher Sue Dumais often says, "Emotions are energy in motion." They are meant to move, not be buried inside. If we never look directly at our fears, we may miss something that can dramatically affect our perspective on life and our emotional wellbeing.

To Practise This

To practise this in your own life, sit in a quiet space with your eyes closed. Imagine that your crown chakra at the top of your head is open. See or feel a large funnel of light and love entering the top of your head and washing over you. Now bring your awareness either to your root chakra at the base of your spine or to the soles of your feet (if they are planted on the floor). Welcome a grounding cord of energy that connects you to the earth. Feel the magnetic, loving connection between you and the earth.

Now ask Spirit: "Please show me what I am afraid to see or know. Thank you. Thank you."

Sit patiently, allowing an image or knowingness to present itself. Once you have received this information, allow yourself to dip into the feeling that is present. Permit yourself to fully feel whatever is there. You are safe to feel the sadness or fear. Feel it and allow it to express itself. You might experience tears or a slight trembling. Let it move up and out of your body. Remember to breathe.

If you aren't shown any images or don't feel anything, be gentle with yourself and try again at another time. If you have experienced trauma, you may want to work together with an experienced healer.

Stress-Free Decisions

Should I quit my job? Should I move to a new city? Should I leave my spouse? Should I break up with my business partner? Should I learn a new profession? Should I accept a better-paying job? Decisions, decisions, decisions.

Fear of making the "wrong" decision can shoot a person's stress up to the moon. The pressure to make the "right" decision can spike our anxiety, leaving us sleepless and confused. Around and around and around we go, riding the merry-go-round of our mind. Overanalyzing and neurotic. All-consuming, it's hard to focus on anything else. Frightened to make a mistake. Afraid to miss an opportunity. We have all been there.

Big decisions used to stress me out. I repeatedly compared the pros and cons of each decision. I would lie awake at night, filled with anxiety and fear. When we assume that it is entirely our responsibility to make decisions in our life, the pressure to make the "right" decision can feel overwhelming.

However, when we begin to trust that Spirit is always guiding us, and the Divine has a grand plan for our life, making decisions becomes stress-free. When we tune into our heart, rather than listen to our overanalyzing, fear-based mind, we begin to hear whispers and feel nudges that we might have otherwise missed. In other words, think less and feel more.

Let Spirit Absorb Your Dilemma

When I was in my early forties, I was blown away to discover that I was pregnant. As the parents of two beautiful daughters, my husband and I had no plan to have a third child. I love babies. I enjoy pregnancy. I knew, if it was meant to be, I could do it again. With some logistical changes, we could make it work. My husband, however, saw the situation as being very black and white. He was not going to have another baby and that was that. But abortion was not something that I considered an option at this stage of my life. I went to bed that night feeling confused, hurt, and alone. Until, that is, I remembered to hand my dilemma over to Spirit.

As I lay in the dark with my head on my pillow, I imagined tossing my situation upwards in a beautiful ball of light for Spirit to absorb and hold. I prayed to be given a clear sign as to how to proceed. And then, I fell asleep peacefully.

In the midst of the early morning darkness, I awoke abruptly. A clear, confident voice rang out in my head: "Make the appointment." I was startled by the message and the authoritative voice. Surprisingly, I managed to fall back asleep. Not long afterwards, I awoke again in the dark. The same crystal clear message sounded in my head: "Make the appointment."

That morning, I found a local clinic and made an appointment. Looking at my calendar, there was only one day and time that would work ideally with my schedule—Wednesday morning. When the receptionist shared that Wednesday at 8:30

a.m. was the clinic's only availability that week, I knew from a deep place within me that Spirit was guiding me. And without getting lost in my own attachments and fears, I loyally followed the guidance.

Speaking with the clinic nurse during the appointment, I learned that, due to certain symptoms, there was a possibility that my body might miscarry. In awe and gratitude, I burst into tears. The Divine was reassuring me that this baby wasn't part of the grand plan for me and my spouse. Although I intuitively sensed that a third baby was not meant to be, this decision would have been far too emotionally challenging for me to make on my own.

By handing the situation over to the Divine and asking Spirit to show me my next step, I took myself out of the decision-making equation. After all, it really wasn't my decision to make. In fact, none of our life decisions are meant to be made alone in our conscious minds. Instead, we are meant to follow the guidance and go with the flow.

To Practise This

To practise this in your own life, sit or lie in a quiet space. Imagine that you are placing your dilemma or your decision into a ball of light. Then see yourself gently tossing the ball upwards for the Universe to hold. Now trust that the Universe can orchestrate a solution. Trust that you will be given clear guidance and shown your next step.

Now ask Spirit: "Please hold this situation for me. I understand that this dilemma or decision is not for me to figure out. Please give me a clear sign. Show me how to proceed. Thank you, thank you."

Nature, the Relaxation Jackpot

Spending time in nature has been one of my trusted, stress-busting techniques for many years. Thankfully (but not coincidentally), I live within steps of numerous green parks and a short walk to the ocean and beaches. When I feel anxious, agitated, or confused, I head outside to walk, to jog, or simply to sit. Relaxing on the beach and soaking up the calming, powerful energy of the expansive ocean does wonders for my mood and wellbeing. Like the change that comes with the flip of a light switch, my mood shifts automatically from irritable and anxious to optimistic and relaxed.

The beauty and power of nature helps me put my life into perspective. Instantaneously, the issues that I perceived as problems shrink in size, sometimes even completely vanishing. Anxiety and worry slip away. When I'm in nature, my heart fills with gratitude and love. I can feel my alignment with our all-loving Source and my connection with our beautiful earth.

Exposure to nature has been shown to calm people. A *National Geographic* article titled "This is Your Brain on Nature" shares several research results on the stress-lowering effect of nature. In 2009, Dutch researchers found a lower rate of fifteen diseases (including anxiety and depression) in people who lived within about 800 metres (approximately half a mile) of green space. In a Japanese study, eighty-four subjects walked through various forests for fifteen minutes, while the same number of people strolled around a city. Researchers discovered that those who walked among the trees experienced a 16 percent decrease in cortisol, our body's stress hormone.

To Practise This

To practise this in your life, hop on your bike, lace up your shoes, rent a kayak, or grab your skis. Sit in a flower-filled garden or relax on the beach and breathe in the ocean. Whatever calls to you. Feel inspired by the miracle of nature.

Life Is Happening *for* You

Life is scattered with events and circumstances that can trigger anxiety and other uncomfortable emotions. These challenges are really gems in disguise—opportunities to grow and heal. We can be curious about our responses to life. Ask yourself, "Do I repeatedly experience feelings of anxiety, anger, distrust, loneliness, or helplessness? Do I notice myself feeling unheard, unloved, or unworthy?" Sometimes it can feel as if life is happening to us and we are powerless victims. This is however not true. As Sue Dumais teaches, "Life is happening FOR you." The Universe is orchestrating events for our healing.

Don't waste time looking outside yourself for who is to blame or what is not right in your life. Commit to looking within and allowing yourself to feel what is there in your heart. Feel the emotion in its entirety. And let it go. Keeping your emotions buried and hidden is like walking in circles in a dark forest. It might feel familiar and therefore somewhat safe because you recognize the same trees and the same boulders, but, if you stay there, you will never experience the joy of feeling the warmth and light of the radiant sun and the expansiveness of an open meadow filled with wildflowers.

I now let go of the anxious need to control my outward experiences. I trust that Spirit is guiding me, and the Divine has my back. By regularly handing over decisions and dilemmas to a higher power, I am able to loosen my anxious grip on the steering wheel that directs my life. The more I let go of control and trust that Spirit is guiding me, the more I am able to go with the flow and relish the awe-inspiring scenery along my journey.

In the past, I looked at life through the filter of anxiety. Today, I am able to experience life from a softer and calmer place. As I've illustrated in this chapter, some of my anxiety and fear stemmed from past-life events, while much of my stored feelings were picked up on while in utero and during early childhood. I've learned to see and trust the perfection of the Divine's plan for my life. I believe that we choose our parents. It was predetermined that my mom and I would be in a close mother-daughter relationship. My mom has played her role perfectly. She has helped teach me the lessons I am here to learn, allowing me to expand and evolve.

Embracing the Healer Within

For many years, I have been aware of a gentle force pulling me along my path, awakening me, and showing me how I am meant to be of service in this wonderful, crazy world.

In January 2015, I began training as an intuitive healer with Sue Dumais. In December 2015, I became one of Heart Led Living's first Certified Intuitive Healers. During the past three years, I have further honed my skills in the advanced mentoring program. Working with the images and feelings that flood me when I tune into an individual's energy, I am able to help clients shine light on and release stored emotions and buried fears. I thank the Divine for my intuitive gifts and for allowing me to help people to access their own innate joy and freedom. Being of service as a clear channel fills my heart and offers me a deep sense of purpose and peace.

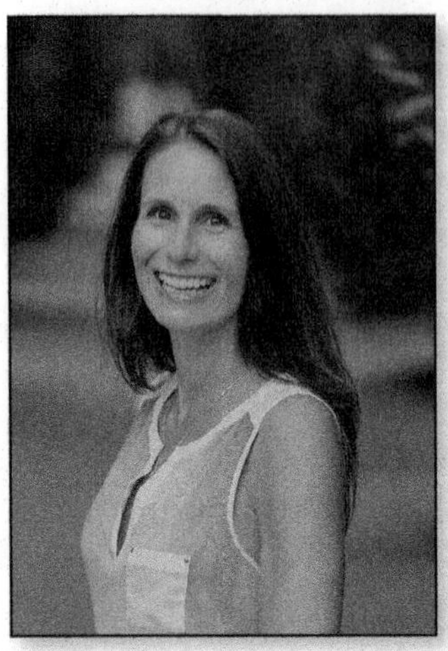

Author Biography for Rachel Shoniker, Entrepreneur, Writer, and Certified Intuitive Healer

Born in Ontario, Canada, Rachel Shoniker moved with her parents several times before the young family settled down in a pristine mountain town in the Interior of British Columbia. To the outside world, Rachel's life appeared to be sprinkled with various accomplishments and niceties. Unfortunately, her inner world tainted how she felt about herself and her life. No matter what she accomplished or how highly others perceived her, a gnawing, toxic anxiety left her breathless and in a constant state of panic, fear, and self-doubt.

At thirty years of age, Rachel had a startling epiphany. Not only did she not like herself, she loathed herself. With this shocking awareness, her healing journey had officially begun. Her quest to feel peace and happiness placed her on a spiritual path that offered her profound personal transformations and unexpectedly revealed her gift as a clairvoyant. Along the way, Rachel developed a deep trust in the perfection of the Divine's plan. She learned to go with the flow, rather than pushing, stressing, and striving.

In December 2015, Rachel became one of Heart Led Living's first Certified Intuitive Healers. During the past three years, Rachel has continued to hone her skills as an intuitive healer in Heart Led Living's advanced mentoring program. Working with the images and feelings that flood her when she tunes into an individual's energy, she helps clients shine light on their stored emotional hurt and buried fears, thereby allowing them to access their own innate joy, freedom, and peace.

Rachel lives with her husband and two beautiful daughters in downtown Vancouver, where she relishes being near the city's beaches, ocean, green parks, and mountains. To learn more about Rachel and her offerings, visit www.heartledliving.com/our-coaches/rachel-shoniker/.

Chapter 6

I Asked "WHY ME?" and Got the Answer "Why Not Me?"

by Delle Vaughan

I Asked "WHY ME?" and Got the Answer "Why Not Me?"

by Delle Vaughan

Tibetan Buddhism Firsthand

I lived my life for the first thirty years questioning "Why Me?" around different areas of my life's journey. My biggest lessons have been around my childhood—navigating who I was as opposed to my parents' expectations for me; bringing those expectations into my marriage of thirty-six years; and raising our three sons, only to have to let go and find my own true path. I went through so many life lessons and I see that it was all purposeful and meant to be. Both my husband and I are stronger now having had to grow and heal our inner wounds. We accept each other and also forgave any hurtful or unaware actions that we took. We see that with our own humanness we have raised three amazing sons who are also accepting of their journeys. We realized that after thirty years of being together, we now had to see our marriage in a different light, talk on a different level of awareness, and grow together with the newness that had become our reality.

I travelled through Eastern Asia with my family over a period of a few years and while I was there, I felt an inner sense of peace and calmness. I love how Asians parent; I love the beauty of meditation and mindfulness. I came home and started studying with a Tibetan teacher; I loved the philosophy and awareness that Tibetan Buddhists hold within themselves. I felt the peace in my soul when I read that we choose our parents for a reason each lifetime.

Now, I truly believe we choose our families and definitely our parents. Tibetan Buddhism teaches a belief that we have karmic connections, a son with his mother and a daughter with her father. I can honestly say my journey has been about those karmic connections and the many lessons I have learned by being a daughter and then beautifully being a mother.

Regarding my relationship with my parents and sister, I can see that the lessons I had were all lessons I had to learn in this lifetime. I knew that my sons had chosen me and their dad so that we could see and grow through all of the challenging and humbling lessons we have experienced over the years.

My Childhood

I was raised in a controlling and co-dependent family. We lived a structured life and everything was always so neat and tidy. My mother's love was contingent on my behaving in a certain manner. I was told numerous times during my childhood that she could so easily walk away and never speak to me again. The worry about going against the grain brought with it a huge amount of self-doubt, negative talk, and self-criticism. I never felt I could speak my truth or confront my mother or anyone else on any level or there would be a withdrawal of affection, love, and approval.

I realize now from my experiences that my mom was coming from a place of fear—her own wounds from her childhood. I always knew my mother loved me from her heart but she had times in her life when she wasn't able to maintain that awareness and would go into a place of survival for herself. It was almost as though, if she was able to withhold the power of love and affection, she was then able to remain strong. For years I have questioned my actions around others; I worried about showing my authentic self because I was never good enough as a child. And now I question whether that was what I was told or whether it was an inner belief I attached to as a young child. The feeling of unworthiness was an underlying emotion that was constantly with me.

Meeting My Husband-to-Be

The meeting with my husband was the Universe bringing us together at a time when neither of us was looking or wanting to have a relationship. I was just trying to regain my footing around a relationship that had ended and he was on his way to Australia. Forward a few months, we were engaged and I was going against my family for the first time in my life, but I knew in my heart that he was the man I was to be with.

Life and lessons since have shown that someone higher guided me to share this life path with him. And it has been a path of incredible growth, love, heartache, and change.

I became very independent over the first few years we were

married. I felt a sense of confidence that I hadn't felt before. Within myself I started to feel the immense power of being able to handle my life and our home exactly the way they were meant to be for us.

Yet in the back of my subconscious, I felt I was constantly making excuses for him and for the fact that we made choices that worked for us but didn't fit into the "normalcy" of my family. I was in constant self-judgment about what my family thought and how they would judge us and him. I was never able to stand up and stop the judging at that time as the fear of being cut off and not belonging was greater than finding the independence I so loved and craved. One powerful lesson I have learned over the years is "The fear of the unknown is far greater than the fear of the known." So, for me to make huge life changes, I learned to come from a place of complete inner trust, knowing that I was always supported by a guidance far greater than me. I was married to a man who loved me and believed in me and he never gave me anything but the support and belief that I could do and be anything I wanted to be. It has taken me years to finally believe that within me is what he had always seen.

Listening to My Children and Silencing My Husband

While pregnant with my first child, I had a deep knowing that I was going to have to truly listen, and become aware of any controlling and self-sabotaging traits I had, knowing the impact they would have on my child. It came to me so very clearly that I didn't want to repeat some of the parenting that I had been raised with. I had an inner knowing that this child would be the start to a road of healing for me. Interestingly, this was also the start of a rocky road of letting go of old stories and habits around my birth family.

After the birth of my son, I had such an incredible sense of connection to something greater than me. I have always believed in God, but this was an inner knowing of the miracle of having this child coming into my life's journey. I realized how exhausted I was from keeping all areas of my life together. The Universe started showing me the signs and giving me nudges that I was very resistant to see. I was constantly juggling my husband and my marriage and what we were doing to keep my parents happy. I have to acknowledge that, because of my fear, I wouldn't let my husband be heard. I constantly asked him to walk away to avoid any form of a confrontation with them, so I was also putting a wedge between us. I now realize how dishonouring it was to both of us and to the family we had created together. My voice and inner needs are truly important. I have value in what I want and need to share.

Our second son was born twenty months later and my husband and I had come together closer as a family with my parents. We had seemed to move into a new place of respect and understanding.

We decided that my father would become a partner in our company. I had an inner knowing that this wasn't a decision that would benefit anyone in the long run, but it was also great to finally be putting down the gavel. Unfortunately, as the year went by, tensions escalated and the working arrangement wasn't working. I was pregnant with my third child at this time and I was back into that old pattern of wanting everything to work out with no conflict or confrontation; I was still battling my fear of losing my parents' love. Even though I was now a mother with my own family, this fear was something deeply ingrained in my thinking. As my due date came closer, the business partnership broke down. I was so exhausted and also angry that at this time once again I was dealing with issues that seemed to be a recurring themes in my life. I knew that at some point I would have to step into my true self and make a stand, but at that time the fear of abandonment was still far too great.

Abandonment

Everything seemed to come to an abrupt end the day my youngest son was born. My parents had decided to leave the business and that day my mom made it quite clear she was also willing to walk away from me. I left the hospital, we gathered our other two sons from my parents and we took our three boys home. I have since realized that when we don't look at our past and heal around our own abandonment wounds, they keep showing up in our own life. I saw how my mother was coming from that place within of her deep abandonment wounds. I so dearly loved her, but I wasn't able to heal her; she had to be willing to do the work herself.

The next few weeks were a blur, as I think back on them. Every fear I had ever had came to the forefront in the days that followed my coming home with our third son. The fear of abandonment was huge. Not being able to function as a new mom, I wondered how I could truly care for my young sons when I was walking around in a state of such deep panic.

My husband has always worked out of town for extended periods of time and although he had been home since the birth of our youngest son, he had to head away for what was to be at least a week up in the Northwest Territories. He had only been gone a couple of days when I left my children with a friend for a very brief time. A situation happened during which a trust was broken. I blamed myself.

My initial reaction was one of fear. "I am unworthy of being a parent, a wife." All my childhood beliefs came back to me with a vengeance. My sense of guilt and shame for being "less than" was overwhelming. I truly believed my husband would withdraw his love and I would be alone. Over a period of twenty-four hours, I allowed my ego to completely take over all thoughts of good within myself, replacing them with complete unworthiness in all areas of my life, regarding my parents, my sons, and my husband.

So, when my husband came through the front door the next morning after only being away three days, saying how he had had a strange feeling he needed to come home, I truly saw that the Universe had always been giving me guidance and support but I had never been willing to see it. When I voiced my fear that he would leave me and take our sons away from me he was stunned. He couldn't believe that thought would ever cross my mind.

I had a glimpse of the unconditional love he always has for me and that was the love I knew I would give to my sons. I would not repeat the past of my childhood. I would not be a victim of my life's circumstances, nor would I raise my sons to be victims either. My life had changed. All the years leading up to that point had given me insights, but I never had been willing to listen or change. Now, I was ready.

Starting My Healing

Days later, I opened the phone book and found the name of a homeopathic doctor. I bundled us all up and this was the start of my healing and searching. Dr. Sandhu saved my life that day. I had postpartum depression and was feeling completely adrift. He heard me and started me on the path of healing myself inside and out. What I loved and still love about homeopathic medicine is the wisdom that "What the body creates, the body can heal." I needed help to heal myself mentally and physically, so I could then start the process of healing myself spiritually.

That was a turning point. Incredible people began coming into my life, helping me to heal myself from that time forward.

I met a beautiful woman who was an incredible channel able to share her knowing and knowledge. She passed on a book *Why Me, Why This, Why Now: A Guide to Answering Life's Toughest Questions* by Robin Norwood. I read it and instantly was filled with a sense that I had finally found the beliefs I could resonate with; I was on a road that I knew intuitively would be right. It was the first time I felt as though I could relate to all those years I had said to myself, "There must be more to life than this heartache." I stepped back from old patterns and routines I had been doing. I had an inner knowing that was always present but I had ignored for years because I didn't want to go against "the norm."

I read any and all books that came across my path. Reading *Linking Up: How the People in Your Life Are Road Signs to Self-Discovery* by Catherine Ann Lake brought me to an awareness that everyone comes onto our path for a reason. Some stay, some for a while, others for a short time.

I know that through this whole period of time, the Universe was guiding me in raising our three sons. I had something greater than myself guiding me when I was having to let go of my ego. I let go of what parenting should be like. I would ask them what they were needing and we would then work it out. I tried to honour each of them and their uniqueness.

I will admit I was a hypervigilant mother, as there was still a lingering fear that if I should let my guard down, anything would and could happen. That has probably been one of the longest fears I have carried and I was hesitant to let it go.

I started healing around my birth family and through all of

this I started to have a new awareness around my parents and their actions. They had never come from a place of not loving enough; instead I saw that they were having to walk through their own journey, their own fears and programming from their childhoods, with a lack of awareness and questioning. But through this time of being apart from my parents, my mom especially started opening and healing. My love for her was always so deep within me, but we now became more than mother and daughter—we are truly wonderful friends. Our karmic connection became one of healing and acceptance.

Asking and Receiving Guidance

In 2012 I had my next nudge, thankfully with greater personal awareness. I started seeing shifts in my marriage and my husband. He, who had always been so strong and grounded, was starting to ask the question of "Why am I not happy?" He was tired of his responsibilities and I think he was overwhelmed with the weight of his work and the numerous pressures around it. Even having gone through cancer eight years earlier, he had never taken the time to look within and face any of *his* fears. He did what he did best, which was to dig deeper and work harder and push his emotions a little further inside.

It was also around this time I was starting to see my intuitive self becoming more and more present. I was trying to look at the decisions and actions I was taking by listening and feeling the guidance within me. I remember one day going outside and standing beneath the beautiful old cedar trees we have on our property. I raised my hands to the sky and asked for the message to come in.

The next day, a close friend came over and said, "Delle, open your doors. You have so many spirits trying to come in."

So I smudged my house, opened my doors, and asked for guidance once more. I asked to see what I was to be told. Within a twenty-four-hour period of time, my life completely changed again. My marriage had been betrayed at the deepest level of trust, our business of thirty-two years was in a very precarious state, and we were at the tip of legal issues with a member of my birth family. I could feel the ground giving way under me this time and I experienced the old fears of abandonment and being unworthy coming in. I had some level of awareness that at times felt as though I was standing on the outside looking on as this story unfolded.

My first thought was about myself. What had I missed? What wasn't I listening to or seeing? I felt a pull to go back to my old conditioning as a child and to retreat and hide. I wanted to run away and get out of everything; I didn't want to face my marriage, the business, and even having to be strong for the boys. I was at a point of truly not knowing what to do and I couldn't believe what was happening around me.

It was a close friend who said, "Don't walk away from thirty years of living with a man who is not the person who betrayed you." She said what I was needing to hear at that moment so that I could step back from the old fears and try to be available.

I fell two weeks later and broke my right femur bone at the hip. It was the type of break that happens in a high-impact car accident. As a dear friend said, "It was a rebirth!" The Universe had stopped me in my tracks. I was forced for the first time in my life to be vulnerable. I couldn't do anything for anyone let alone for myself. I couldn't run away. I couldn't look after anyone else. I was forced to be quiet, to lie there, to process my life, and to let all the lessons I had gone through to wash over me. I felt I had been put in a position in which my husband and I had to come together and bring our marriage back to some level of trust and forgiveness.

As I have worked through my pain and deep hurt, I have been able to see the incredible pain and soul changes that have also occurred within my husband. I am humbled at times now to see how the hurt we endured has actually been a gift in allowing both of us to heal. I saw the man to whom I had been married for thirty years—a man who had never expressed his feelings—come to a place of total surrender. I had to let go of my expectations of what a marriage should be and see it for what it is. It is two people walking a journey together with both allowing their shadows within to come up, be looked at, and then released. I allowed forgiveness to come into my being at a core level. My husband has also had to forgive himself and take accountability for his actions. By forgiving himself he has been able to free himself from his old expectations. "Forgiveness is like humility. It is fragile and to speak of it is to lose it."

Time to Walk the Walk

A very close friend told me, "It is now time for you to start walking the walk and stop talking the talk."

With awareness, I saw that all the gems of knowledge and learning I had gathered over the years were leading up to this moment. I had trained and became a Clinical Hypnotherapist and saw the power of the subconscious mind and our beliefs. I re-read papers I had gathered over the years on the lessons we come here to learn. I became aware that my journey has been around releasing expectations and seeing others exactly for who they were. I had been able to do that with my sons and I was and am in awe that I had the strength within me to follow my vision as a mother. I had to look at my parents and sister and, although I had forgiven them years earlier, I was able to see that they are only humans living their journey, walking it in the way that they are able.

I had done a retreat on the Tibetan approach to living and dying just before this and it was as though I had being given all the tools I would need to step up to this level of my life path. I had come out of the retreat looking at the fragility of life and also how we are each here to learn the lessons that come to us, whether they come through self-direction or not. I had to allow myself to let go of my ego and see that I was married to a good man who had made a truly hurtful and life-impacting choice. I had to think and reflect about who he was and what we had together throughout our marriage. I had to find it in my heart to listen to the guidance I was receiving and then forgive him. I wanted to show my sons that anything can be forgiven if there is an honest and genuine acknowledgment, that sometimes family members screw up, but we can move forward if we work and truly step into ownership of our actions.

I had done much work around understanding childhood and seeing how the early years of a child's development can truly mould that child into an adult. I could no longer ask that question of "Why Me?" because, when I stepped back and looked at the events unfolding in my life, I had seen the miracles that come and say, "Why Not You?" I would have never searched nor realized that my journey has been one of looking within, listening to the guidance I am being shown. I have come to see that when I listen to my inner guidance and can hear it clearly, I am always supported. I can also say that the times I have knowingly gone against my guidance, because of ego, I have been let down or made decisions and acted in ways that have impacted me or those I love negatively.

I wouldn't have made good choices to follow my heart

these past few years, if it weren't for the community and other healers who are around me. I have found my connection to a divine source that has always been present and is now a part of my everyday life. I have seen how beautiful life is when there is no judgment around who I am or what I bring forward. I was led to join an inspiring heart led community and, in these past few months, I have felt as though all my years of searching, gathering knowledge, listening to my guidance, and then living through periods of time that were life-changing have brought me here. As my teacher and mentor Sue Dumais has said, "When we resist change, we resist life. When we resist life, life appears to resist us."

I choose to live fully in this life, with a lightness and deep compassion for those I love to carry forward with them. I want to think I have shown my sons it is okay to fall, but we need not be the victim of our life. I would love to think I can reach one woman who is feeling as though she is cut off and floundering with this new responsibility of mothering a new child. I would love her to know that she is not alone and she has all the power and guidance she needs around her and within her, if she is willing to stop and listen.

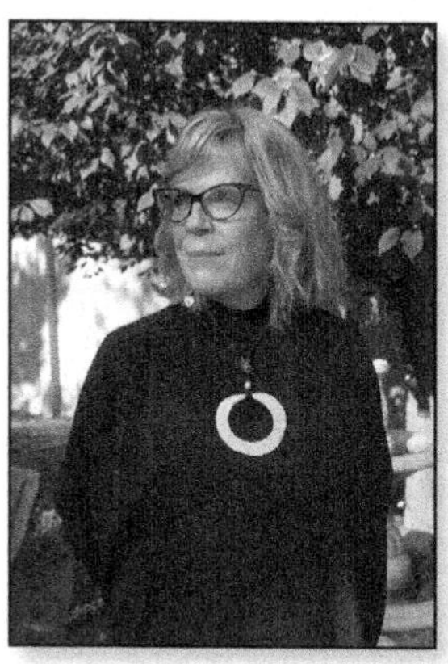

Author Biography for Delle Vaughan, Intuitive Coach, Conscious Parenting Advocate, Craniosacral Therapist

Delle Vaughan is a seeker of life's hardest questions. She is a passionate advocate of conscious parenting and honouring the child even before they are born. She receives inner guidance when working with new mothers to help them to see old patterns and beliefs that they may bring forward into their parenting. She believes that with support and a heart led community, a new awareness around life's hardest questions can be healed. She deeply believes that forgiveness is a journey of letting go of our ego thoughts and being able to see that with forgiveness comes an inner peace. She sees with clarity that we are all here in this lifetime to learn the lessons we have come to learn.

Her belief that everything happens for a reason and that the people who come onto our path have a meaning and a purpose is the main source of strength in her healing and work. She is a clinical hypnotherapist who has also studied to be a holistic birth doula. Delle believes in a baby's incredible open consciousness. Nurturing this provides a strong base for the first years of life, the years when many beliefs, morals, and inner strengths are formed. She believes that we need to live a life of love and compassion for ourself and for the greater consciousness of our community. She believes that by listening to our inner guidance we can align our life with spirit and help in our own inner healing.

Delle is a wife, daughter, sister, and a devoted mother to her three sons and their families. She believes that her children have chosen to walk their journey with her and that the lessons she has learned from them have helped to guide her on her path of life and healing.

Delle lives in Victoria, British Columbia with her husband and their Aussie labradoodle, Dharma.

To learn more about Delle and her offerings, visit dellevaughan.com.

Chapter 7

Holy Shift ~ Divorce is a Gift

by Lisa Windsor

Holy Shift ~ Divorce is a Gift

by Lisa Windsor

The Path of Divorce

Eleven years into my marriage, my Inner Voice said, "Have no more hope ... it will not change." And finally I surrendered and admitted defeat. My marriage had failed and I faced the idea of divorce for the first time. The concept of family that I had constructed in my mind was now going to be deconstructed. My whole life was about to change.

I had married at the age of twenty-two. I never imagined that my marriage would end in divorce eleven years later. My upbringing taught me that the commitment to my marriage was of paramount importance. I learned that a strong couple has early morning coffee together on the weekends and they never go to sleep angry with one another. But right away, there were flaws with that prescription. First off, my husband had no interest in sitting with me on those quiet weekend mornings and second of all, although we tried, we consistently ended up angry at one another when we went to bed at night.

But no worries, I quickly learned that my relationship looked different from my parents' relationship and I adjusted, and adjusted some more, and adjusted even more to try and make the union feel united. I had to loosen from the loyalty and devotion I had for my husband.

In the beginning of my marriage, I had seen him as my provider, protector, and director, but he never did a good job at fulfilling those roles. I suffered a lot of pain and frustration through my marriage and lost my voice. I silently stood by as countless decisions were made that felt out of integrity with my heart. Poor financial decisions and work decisions often caused massive stress and I would do my best to deny the problems and focus instead on the kids. But it was all having a very big impact.

During my marriage my main focus was on expanding my family and building a solid relationship. I was doing a lot of personal development work and I was having babies! Four beautiful babies! My husband and I loved kids and we parented well together. Our children united us and gave us a joint purpose.

During that time, I was training as a Life Coach and Wellness Counsellor and an opportunity for free marriage counselling was presented. Our counsellor was surprised to find that our parenting style worked well but that our personal relationship was strained and disjunctive. I wanted the two of us to fit together and yet no matter what I tried, the relationship was misaligned. I travelled down many avenues in an attempt to "fix" the marriage but it would always return to the same arguments and grievances.

In the end, I had to come out of denial and recognize the deep level of misery I was experiencing. I had tried to push the pain away, ignore the pain, and suppress the pain because I was so afraid to face the truth that had been plaguing my heart—I wanted out of this relationship. I had to accept that our relationship would not change or be "fixed" in the context of a marriage. I felt like my inner light and spirit were dying.

A Course in Miracles

Once I was clear that I was walking the path of divorce, a new vow and promise arose in my awareness. I vowed to use the divorce to heal all fearful patterns, blocks, and limiting beliefs that I held in my mind. I was committed to not repeating this same relationship model again. I was committed to experiencing true freedom. With this prayer, I could begin to expect miracles. I was absolutely open to miracles as I had been a devoted student and teacher of *A Course in Miracles* (ACIM) for many years.

A Course in Miracles is a transformational spiritual path for healing our minds of fear and connecting us with our Loving Inner Teacher, the Holy Spirit. The curriculum of ACIM leads to the goal of inner peace and lasting happiness. It is a practical path for healing our minds of all fear-based beliefs. ACIM is a self-study book that includes a text and a 365-lesson workbook to guide students through a year of study. The course empowers us to use our mind to choose love over fear. Love is real and fear is not. But we do not escape from a thought system of fear on our own. We must connect with the voice for God, the Holy Spirit, and allow ourselves to be guided along the way to peace.

I was committed to applying everything I had learned from the course to the experience of my divorce. I would have to listen and follow the path the Holy Spirit set out and I would have to practise a radical kind of forgiveness that cleared my mind of fearful thoughts and judgments. I had my faith in God and I was learning to trust in miracles.

The "miracle" in *A Course in Miracles* holds a different definition than the miracles we hear of in the world. The miracle in ACIM is a shift in perception from a fearful perspective to a loving point of view. It occurs on the level of the mind, where we shift between two different thought systems—from a thought system of fear (ego) to a thought system of Love (God, Holy Spirit, Higher Self, Inner Teacher). When our mind changes from fear to love, our perceptual worlds change. Miracles are natural and we are all entitled to them. But we have to be willing to play our part in the healing process.

Our part is to recognize that the cause of our problems is in our mind and not outside us. Our part is also to accept that the solution to our problems is in our mind and not outside us. The problem is the ego and the solution is the Holy Spirit. We must use the power of decision to choose the Holy Spirit as our healer and guide. We are only ever in pain and upset when we choose the ego, and we are only ever in peace and joy when we choose the Holy Spirit. Once we recognize that we have made a wrong choice, we can ask our higher self for help and support. We can open to receiving the miracle that brings a new way of seeing. At first, I viewed my divorce as a failure but when I was willing to heal this perception, I was shown that my divorce was a path to freedom. This change in perspective allowed me to open to the many gifts that divorce would bring.

My Own Intuitive Channels

I didn't know many people who had been divorced and I didn't have anyone close to me that had gone through the process with young children. I was going to need a lot of help and support navigating this new pathway. I had practised *A Course in Miracles* long enough to know that the real support I needed was not external to me. I had to turn inward and place my focus and attention on the Holy Spirit. I had been developing a relationship with the Holy Spirit over a few years and was really learning to trust that I could follow his guidance.

The Holy Spirit communicates differently and more expansively than the way people communicate. He spoke to me through my own intuitive channels. Directions came to me in inner visions, loving thoughts, and inspired ideas. I saw signs and noticed synchronistic events. The Holy Spirit spoke to me through people, music, and movies. *Under the Tuscan Sun* is an inspiring film I watched about one woman's journey through divorce. As I watched it, I placed the Holy Spirit in charge of my mind so I could receive His perspective on the film. I saw how the main character learned to follow her heart by opening to the many signs and symbols placed on her path for her healing and happiness. She shed many tears, took many risks, and walked right through the mess to the sunshine and peace that lay beyond. My heart stirred with joy and hope, and reminded me that I was not alone and that the Holy Spirit would reveal each step necessary for my own healing. I was learning that the Holy Spirit's communication resonated in my heart, had a peaceful quality, and was always certain.

Along with teaching Inner Guidance, *A Course in Miracles* teaches forgiveness as the pathway to healing. Again, it does not use the world's usual definition of "forgiveness" but a radical form of forgiveness that instructs us to take every fearful thought, every difficult situation, and every relationship to the Holy Spirit for a healed perception. I had a daunting job ahead of me with the divorce. It felt like my whole life had been picked up, shaken apart, and left in an enormous mess.

I felt like an immovable mountain of chaos stood before me, holding my life in total disarray. To clean my life up seemed impossible but I knew the power of Love (God) was within me and the Holy Spirit would direct me. I gathered my courage to face the mountain of mayhem. I had faith in miracles and I had trust in the Holy Spirit.

What If?

My now-ex-husband and I had a lot to sort out when we first separated, but it was clear in the beginning that we would set up a plan to share and be responsible for the kids equally. I remember the first time the kids stayed with their dad, leaving me alone. When I was on my own, it didn't take long for a cluster of fearful thoughts to surface. "What if I have made a giant mistake? How will I survive? What if I'm wrong?" This is what it sounded like when the ego was in charge in my mind. The thoughts would whirl and circulate over and over in relentless patterns.

I happened to be housesitting for my sister that evening so I headed to her place with terror rising in my mind. I lay in bed and was paralyzed. I was so afraid to turn within because I feared the worst. "What if I messed my whole life up?"

I was guided to a deck of spiritual cards that my sister kept for receiving messages from the Divine. I took a deep breath and reached for a card in the deck. I sat for one … two … three minutes, feeling very afraid to read the message. When I finally had the courage to turn it over, I was shocked by what I read. "Problem resolved." I felt tremendous gratitude and relief and was ready to surrender and turn inward. There I experienced some of the deepest peace I had ever felt. True inner peace … inside and out.

The Holy Spirit did not waste time in unwinding my mind from the fearful patterns and unhealthy interactions I had created with my ex-partner. *A Course in Miracles* was also having a big impact and I was learning that God, being my Source, is my true provider, protector, and director. The Holy Spirit was helping me find my voice again.

To begin, I had to learn to say "no." During my marriage, I believed that fulfilling my role as a good wife meant saying "yes" to the majority of my husband's requests. When we separated and my ex-partner asked for help, I was directed by my inner wisdom to say "no." Over and over again, whether he asked me to pick up something from the store or he wanted to change plans with the kids without notice, I faced the difficult task of denying simple requests and appearing very unhelpful. It was essential that I turn to the Holy Spirit to communicate with my ex-husband, because I had no idea how to unwind from the pattern of people-pleasing and partner-pleasing I had been practising for so long. On my own, I didn't know the answer but with the Holy Spirit's guidance, I was learning to discern between a true "yes" and a true "no."

It took over a month before I received from the Holy Spirit my first "yes" to my ex-husband's request. He had asked if the kids could stay with me for two extra days and I told him I would check in and let him know. In a quiet moment, I turned within and asked the Holy Spirit for clarity. I received a vision of love exploding like fireworks. The answer was "yes!"

My fear to ask within and communicate the Holy Spirit's answer to my ex-husband had fallen away and I received the miracle. I was now aligning with my inner wisdom in my communication with my ex-partner. My ex-partner was learning not to rely on me and I was learning not to take care of him. Old patterns were being undone and I was feeling free to speak my truth.

"Returning to My Father's House"

Once separated, I was guided to move in with my parents and return to the home I had grown up in. My parents had retired and yet had decided to stay in our childhood home, just in case I or my sisters ever needed a place to stay. I actually used to laugh about this, telling them it was silly to keep a big home for just the two of them. I never imagined that I would be the one they had kept the house for! I'm sure my parents had many fears as their household of two grew to a household of seven, but they kept a very positive outlook and made us feel welcome. I was thankful for the half-time set-up with the kids that I had arranged with my ex-partner, because it allowed my parents to experience both a busy, bustling household with their grandchildren and also a quiet, spacious household to relax and stretch out.

Our new home was a tremendous gift and the Holy Spirit communicated that through a beautiful symbol. The day we moved in was Thanksgiving Day! I couldn't help but feel gratitude for my parents' generosity and this cozy setting that enveloped us. It was part of the Holy Spirit's plan to reassure me that I was loved and safe. The Holy Spirit also shared the message that I was "Returning to my father's house." This move was truly representing my return home to God and the awareness of his all-encompassing love. My childhood home became a safe sanctuary for me and my kids, a place where I could face the messy process of divorce.

I was reassured by the Holy Spirit that this divorce was

going to be best for the kids. I was shown that the marriage had deteriorated to the point where the kids were really on the sidelines. As we kept trying to fix the marriage, we were less present and attentive as parents. Once on my own, I felt more available as a mom. The kids were ages nine, seven, four, and two, and I felt that the Holy Spirit was helping me to develop greater patience as a parent and to communicate a message of love and safety to them during this transitional time. The kids did remarkably well through the process. Each of them has been able to express grief and disappointment in the family not staying together and each has also come to see the gifts of their new life routine. They have settled into their two homes and they move peacefully back and forth greeting me with hugs every few days and leaving me with hugs as well.

The arrival at my parents' home also brought a lot of clarity and healing. I could look upon things with greater perspective and hear the Holy Spirit's voice more easily. A beautiful message came to me that first evening. I was told, and felt it in the depth of my being, that leaving my marriage was the single most powerful act of self-love I had ever experienced. I had freed myself from worldly promises so that the promise of my heart to listen and follow God's direction and be at peace could be fulfilled. I was committed more than ever to follow my heart and accept the gifts of God's love. I felt true love toward myself. I was saving myself from the hell of moving in direct opposition to my heart.

To learn true love for self, I was given these instructions: "Good, bad, or ugly … love yourself through it." I was going to learn to love myself from the inside out. I had shown up for the greatest assignment of my life—I had come to love myself, know myself as love, and forgive myself for all the mistakes of my past.

I was guided to create a list dividing the furniture between me and my ex-partner. I didn't really understand at the time but, on paper, the list looked a lot better in his favour than in mine. I would get the kids' bedroom furniture and my office furniture and half of the kitchen possessions. He would get virtually everything else. Because my parents' home was already furnished, I would need a storage unit for the boxes and furniture I was bringing along.

My dad had bought a new boat and it was parked on one side of his garage. When I was waiting for clarity about storage and worrying about the monthly cost, my dad decided that he would park his boat permanently up country where they holiday and he gifted me that half of the garage to store my things. This was the perfect amount of space to store the items I was inspired to bring. The garage was packed floor to ceiling and I was so grateful for this most generous offer. Where I perceived an obstacle or problem, a gift was received instead. The miracle cleared every problem I perceived. I was learning to trust that a peaceful outcome was assured and the answer would be revealed in perfect time. I was developing patience and remembering that trust would solve every problem now.

Learning to Be Alone

Part of my path to experiencing self-love was learning to be alone. This brought up the fear of loneliness. In *A Course in Miracles* we are taught that we are never alone. In fact, it teaches that if we knew who walked with us we would never be fearful again! I was opening up to the Holy Spirit as my most trusted friend, but I was also used to being in a relationship.

When my kids were with their dad, the house became very quiet and my parents invited me often to join them in the evenings for movies. But I had been living apart from my parents for over thirteen years and I felt more inclined to head up to my room for quiet time and reflection.

I remember facing the staircase that led to my room and feeling sure that a stabbing pain of utter loneliness would come to grip me. But the presence of the Holy Spirit was in my mind and he always knew my prayer for love and joining. I would sit up in bed and before I could feel any sense of loneliness I would feel a tangible energy of love hugging and embracing me. I felt as though I was being wrapped in a blanket of love. It was impossible to feel alone! I felt loved and held and remembered! This experience happened multiple times for the first couple of months when I was settling into my new home. I was so grateful for God's love and his constant lesson that he is present in my mind and life.

The Holy Spirit was teaching me that I could trust his guidance. I was learning that I am wholly provided for and cared for. All of the details would be handled and, if I stayed attuned to my inner teacher and remembered to trust, the process would be much gentler. I was learning that each problem I encountered would clear away in perfect time and the miracle would be revealed. Practical matters like dividing assets and possessions as well as sorting out financial matters were included in the healing process.

Learning to Rely on the Holy Spirit

Lesson 50 in A Course in Miracles says "I am sustained by the Love of God." In essence that means that everything we need to follow our highest path for healing and awakening is given to us. In fact, we are wholly provided for and completely taken care of. I wanted to believe this idea but I had always seen my husband as the means by which I was sustained financially. During the separation I became very attached to the home we owned together, hoping that I would be sustained for a while by the proceeds from the sale of the house. I didn't realize I had moved from faith in my husband to faith in this real estate. What a wake-up call I had when we received notice from our city that the home we owned was deemed "high risk" for landsliding. It was built on a fairly steep ravine and the city was now bringing in geotechnical engineers to do a full-scale risk assessment. With this black mark on our property, we were unable to list our home for sale and were told that we might have to build a massive retaining wall the length of the property at the back to reinforce the structure. I was sick with worry as I realized I had put my faith once again in something outside myself and in an instant the home had lost its value and become a liability. I felt like I had nothing left and nowhere safe to look in the world for sustenance.

I was becoming reliant on the Holy Spirit to direct my healing because the life I had known and the things I had owned were all disappearing rapidly. I had nothing to hold on to. I turned inward toward the Holy Spirit to ask for help and support in seeing the situation differently. For the first time, I was going to find out if I was truly sustained by the love of God. I had always felt that I had safety nets in place to catch me if I fell ... but my backup plan had dissolved.

As the months passed, I was learning to live without the external symbols of security. I was developing a deeper trust in the Holy Spirit's plan and feeling an inner security strengthen. *A Course in Miracles* teaches that only God's plan for awakening will work and it emphasizes that our plan will not! God's plan unfolds moment to moment as each component and detail reveals itself in perfect time. I had no control over when this real estate problem would be resolved but I felt encouraged to use this situation for forgiveness.

Finally, the assessment report for the house was completed and in summary there was no real risk of our home landsliding down the ravine. That was a relief, but we were still faced with a major obstacle. By law, when selling a home, everything about the house has to be disclosed to the public, including the reports that had been published about the landslide risk. Even though the house was cleared as safe, there were two reports that remained on the books. The first marked the house as "high risk for landslides" and the second cleared the issue but was written by geotechnical engineers and was not understandable in layman's terms. Our realtor was pessimistic about the chance of a fair sale. The Holy Spirit assured me, "There is no obstacle and no problem," even though, it looked like there was a huge issue standing before us.

We had multiple offers after our first showing but we had not yet disclosed the report. Those four offers fell apart within twenty-four hours. I couldn't believe it. I had to hold faith and absolute trust for the miracle. I would consistently bring my fearful thoughts to the Holy Spirit to clear my anxiety and remember my faith. Two weeks later, we had an offer on the house once again. The sale went through with ease and grace. I learned that the couple who bought the house were engineers and the husband was specifically a geotechnical engineer. He had read the report and understood that the house checked out. What an incredible miracle that the homeowners had the eyes to see that there was no problem! I needed miracle-minded buyers with a higher perspective and that's who showed up! I was learning that I was sustained by my faith in God and reaching peace through this process of forgiveness.

Child Support

There were many lessons around money. I was told by my loving teacher that I would always have the money and resources I needed to follow my heart and take care of my kids. I was learning that I could trust I was cared for and observed that each month I had enough to pay my parents the rent and to cover my basic expenses. For the first time in my life, I clipped coupons and felt inspired to shop at thrift stores. Everything in life simplified. I had fewer possessions and I had to be mindful about every dollar I spent, but I also felt a sense of abundance. I was learning that abundance is a state of mind and has nothing to do with external circumstances.

Even with the Holy Spirit's assurance, insecurities ran deep in my beliefs about lack and financial insecurity. During the legal proceedings of the divorce, I hit a wall of fear when we were trying to sort out child-support payments. I had not worked during our marriage and was attached to being independent and living on my own. I had an amount of child support that I wanted to receive monthly from my ex-husband, but he was suggesting a much lower amount. Every time he mentioned the amount he thought was fair, I became triggered, angry, and scared.

During my marriage, my husband had been the primary breadwinner. I had very little to do with our money and the decisions around spending. I did not agree with how he handled money, but I didn't feel like I had a voice since he was the one earning the income. During the divorce, I would receive money from him when he felt like it. I felt reliant on someone whom I couldn't trust. I wanted my freedom and independence and felt so vulnerable and insecure. I was stuck in a judgmental frame of reference, which was the ego's wrong-minded thinking. But I was still too scared to question my point of view. I wanted to be right at the price of my happiness.

A Course in Miracles teaches that we must drop our defenses to experience true peace.

One particular day, I was rehashing my story of unfairness and entitlement when all of a sudden, I became the witness to the story and realized how tired I was of hearing my own complaints and fear. I was ready to let the story go, even though I did not have a resolution. I was ready to be wrong about it and open up to the Holy Spirit's Guidance. I wanted peace! I was ready to trust!

The Holy Spirit shared a message with me in that moment. "You have been equating your own self-worth with the amount of child support you believe you should receive. Your worth has nothing at all to do with the amount of financial support you will receive. Nothing!"

What I heard resonated truly in my heart. I came home and looked up what "worth" means from the perspective of *A Course in Miracles*. It assured me that my worth was wholly established in God and that nothing could ever change it. I was assured that the ego places our worth on a value scale and we suffer as our sense of self-worth goes lower or higher depending on outside circumstances. My true worth is changeless. I am an innocent and loved child of God.

I surrendered my attachment to my story and gently the Holy Spirit's guidance came to light. I was told that the amount of child support my ex-husband was suggesting was the amount I was to agree to. This meant that for the time being, I could not move from my parents' house and I was uncertain about my future. But I was reassured that I was moving toward greater freedom and it was in my best interests to feel more independent and less reliant on my ex-husband as my life moved forward. I was learning the lesson that I was sustained by the love of God. I was learning to entrust my finances to the wisdom of the Holy Spirit.

In the months and years that have followed, these circumstances inspired me to commit wholly to God's plan. The word "sustainable" would often come to mind and, slowly, the Holy Spirit began revealing a plan for my sustainability that has allowed me to be more independent and less reliant on my ex-husband. My sustainability comes from teaching and sharing about *A Course in Miracles* and inspiring others to turn toward their inner wisdom as a guide to healing and happiness. I call this full-circle healing when my lessons are then used for the highest good of all ... to support and inspire others to trust the Love of God.

Leaving the Details to the Holy Spirit and Forgiving

The miracle I experienced about child support created a huge shift in how I was perceiving the divorce. By surrendering the judgments and grievances held within the old story, I was able to receive the miracle of new perception. The Holy Spirit is an amazing teacher who used every circumstance to reveal a gift of healing. He showed me that I was misusing my mind when I allowed egoic fear-based thinking to dominate my experience. I was learning that when I felt out of control, confused, or angry, it was my thinking that was the problem. My thoughts were out of control. My thoughts were confused. My thoughts were angry.

That day a radical assignment from my loving self came to mind: I was to observe and catch myself anytime I was thinking about my ex-husband or the divorce. These thoughts became a red flag or alert that I had chosen wrongly, that I had chosen fear over love. This was a radical assignment because all of my conditioning had taught me that thinking, analyzing, and sorting out problems is the responsible thing to do. Not only that, I was also afraid that nothing would ever get sorted out if I didn't spend time worrying and troubleshooting all the outstanding issues of my divorce. The Holy Spirit assured me that I was taken care of and that I could rest in faith and trust that everything would be healed in divine time.

This may seem strange, but I was actually concerned about who I was or what my life looked like if I wasn't judging and condemning my ex-husband. So much of my time and energy had been consumed by trying to figure out the divorce and now I was aware that this was no longer helpful. Another part of me was excited to experience the freedom of not having to sort out my life and problems. And I really wanted to discover if, in fact, the Holy Spirit would show up and deliver on his promise.

This is where I was developing courage and patience. It takes courage to be patient! It takes trust to wait for inspired action. In the in-betweens, so much fearful thinking would rise up and this is where the practice of true forgiveness was so helpful. I had to give my mind a job to do. For most of my life, my ego had taken the lead and directed my life and now I was asked to stop listening to the ego and instead forgive. I have to admit, this job is not as prestigious as thinking we are figuring things out and thinking we have the answers, but it was a powerful exercise in learning to be humble and learning to be loved.

So that is what I did; each time I found myself whirling in thoughts of the divorce, I directed the thoughts upward to the Holy Spirit. I would recognize that I had chosen to think ego thoughts and I was ready to hand them upwards to the Holy Spirit for healing. The Holy Spirit gave me a visual for this. He said to imagine I was holding a plate and he was holding a plate. Ego thinking and upset were always on my plate and I would feel stress and heaviness. He would ask me to look at what I had on my plate and when I felt ready to let it go, I could place the thoughts, problems, and situations on his plate for forgiveness. Everything was "for-giving" to the Holy Spirit.

My divorce brought up my greatest fears and even though many of them didn't manifest in form, the fearful beliefs would surface consciously in my mind causing emotional turmoil such as depression, anxiety, and panic. It was a strange process to realize that someone I loved and felt so committed to now appeared as my enemy on an opposing team. I used to trust him to have my back and be there when I needed him. Now, we were quite afraid of one another. I faced fears of lack, fears of not surviving, fears of losing my kids, fears of losing all my money, fears of homelessness, fears of not being good enough, fears of being a failure, feelings of unworthiness, feelings of terror, and a feeling of vulnerability and being out of control. These fears are at the core of the ego-thought system and I knew that they all must eventually come to surface in my awareness in order for me to heal. The divorce was giving me a lot of opportunity to clear my mind of these false perceptions and to purify my mind of fearful beliefs.

Now instead of hanging out in fears of insecurity and frustration, I could practise placing those thoughts and feelings on the Holy Spirit's plate. I was no longer hiding the negative thinking and upset in the dark corners of my mind or shelving the anger for later. I felt empowered to work with my inner teacher to heal my mind.

Receiving the Gifts

A Course in Miracles was teaching me that the remedy to all forms of fear is perfect love. The Holy Spirit represents this perfect love inside my mind. I had found the remedy I had so long been seeking. Pockets of peace were present through much of my divorce because I was practising true forgiveness. I could purify my mind of hatred and fear if I was willing to give all unloving thoughts to the Holy Spirit. He was the perfect purifier of my mind, dissolving what wasn't loving and keeping what was! How perfect! The miracle that was left was love's perception and it always shone a light on the situation and resolved it perfectly, not in my timing but in divine timing.

I was so blessed to have the Holy Spirit as my guide through my divorce. He had taught me "Good, bad, or ugly … love yourself through it." I was shocked at all the ugliness I had to face throughout the process. I really got to see how faith in the ego results in a mind full of attack thoughts. The unconscious fear and guilt that rose up showed me hateful thoughts, jealous thoughts, comparison thoughts, deceitful thoughts, betrayal thoughts, greedy thoughts … so much ugliness. But that experience has also translated into a miracle because I now counsel and teach about true forgiveness and stand as a compassionate witness to others who are ready to expose the ego thoughts rising in their minds.

I know that anything can be healed with the remedy of love. I know that the Holy Spirit is waiting with infinite patience to join with each of us in our minds to help us. He is literally in our minds and available in every moment to extend the support we need to liberate ourselves from fear and to experience true inner peace. I know that I could never be where I am in my life today without God's unceasing love and support. I am forever grateful and beaming with excitement with the idea that God's gifts are for every one of us, if we choose to open up and follow him.

Through my divorce, I faced what I thought was an impassible, impossible mountain of fear. Today, I can say that the mountain has disappeared and the problems of the divorce have been resolved. *A Course in Miracles* was an extraordinary support through this transition. It taught me to trust in the Holy Spirit as my guide and to bring all perceived problems and obstacles to him for a new way of seeing. Through the practice of true forgiveness, I saw many grievances turn to gifts. I received the gift of self-love and the gifts of peace and tranquility. My relationships with my children and parents deepened. Much of the judgment I had for my ex-husband washed away and I was able to free him to live his life on his terms. I have the incredible gifts of my four children as reminders of the eternal love and blessings from my marriage. I am free to follow the path of my heart and continue to trust I am sustained by the Love of God.

I uncovered my true voice and I share the incredible teachings of *A Course in Miracles* to help inspire others to follow the path of their inner wisdom and experience the gifts and miracles that come when we set inner peace as our one goal.

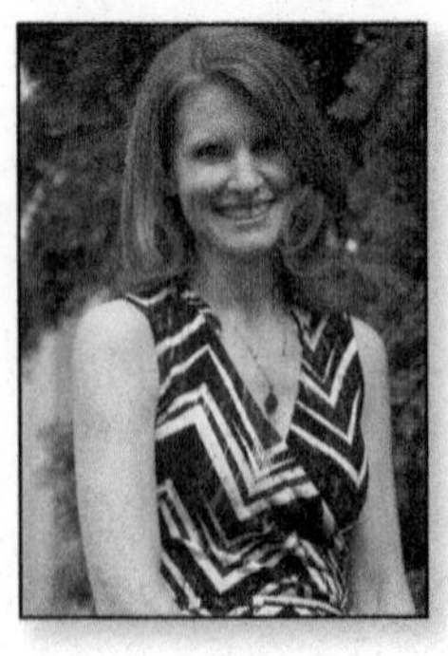

Author Biography for Reverend Lisa Windsor, Founder of Modern Miracles Community

Lisa Windsor earned her Bachelor of Arts in Sociology from the University of British Columbia and went on to become a certified Life Coach and Wellness Counsellor. She co-founded Family Passages Mind-Body Studio and the Heart Led Living Community with her lifelong friend, Sue Dumais. And still, she had not quite answered the call of her heart until she turned her focus to the passion she felt for the transformational teachings of *A Course in Miracles.*

Lisa's love and devotion for *A Course in Miracles* was the catalyst for becoming an Ordained Minister in 2007. She developed a deep trust in her inner teacher as she committed to healing in all areas of her life. Lisa faced many challenges through an eleven-year marriage and with faith and trust she moved through a turbulent divorce. With four young children and her faith in God, Lisa became even more inspired by the profound peace and healing that came from practising true forgiveness and following inner guidance.

Lisa is inspired to share the joyful message that we are loved, whole ,and eternally safe. Her approach is focused on practical application and open-hearted honesty. Through the teachings of A Course in Miracles , Lisa reveals the miracles that occur when we follow our inner guidance and truly forgive.

Lisa lives near Vancouver, British Columbia, with her four amazing kids who inspire her to forgive often and love unconditionally. Her devotion and love of *A Course in Miracles* as inspired her to create the Modern Miracles Community through which she offers spiritual counselling, teaches about *A Course in Miracles*, and facilitates a Certified Minister Training Program.

To learn more about Lisa Windsor and the Modern Miracles Community, visit modernmiracles.ca.

Chapter 8

Black and White to Rainbow

by Kirsty Peckham

Black and White to Rainbow

by Kirsty Peckham

My First Memory of a Miracle

For the longest time I never believed in miracles. Miracles happen every day; we just don't see them.

I'd like to share with you the first memory of a miracle that I recall. It changed the course of my life. I received an email from a new girlfriend, Rachel, saying, "I've got a bit of a crush on you." I was walking my dog and I stopped under a tree to read the message that came through on my phone. It was a turning point. I had to honour it. No second guessing it. It was not part of my plan. It was not how it was meant to be.

The culture I'd been raised in would not see this relationship as traditional. We worked together and had experienced a connection the moment we met. We enjoyed one another's company and could discuss the surface level and deeper aspects of life. I also felt a lot of fear as, at this time in my life, this was taking me off-course, yet I knew this was where I was being taken and I was open to a new way of being and open to the challenge. The moment is carved into my memory—me, the tree, my dog, and the message. My heart actually fluttered. I was alive.

At that point I was in a relationship with Brett my boyfriend of fourteen years and we were trying for a baby; I was on my fertility journey. I had had some in vitro fertilization (IVF) treatments and I'd made lots of practical changes such as improving my diet nutritionally. I was cleaning up my life; if something wasn't good for me, I was dropping it. It was a rollercoaster of a journey.

Rachel and I had become friends very quickly. There was nothing wrong. Perhaps it might have been easier if there was. I had read a blog post by Tosha Silver that describes living life in a comfy prison. That's no way to live a life. I had a clear realization: I needed to tell this woman I was in love with her and I needed to tell my boyfriend that I loved him, but I wasn't "in love" with him. My Soul was speaking now—quietly yet clearly!

Did I want to be living a lie? Lies hurt and I didn't want to hurt.

My Fertility Journey

My fertility journey did several things. It cleaned up my intentions; it taught me how to deal with disappointment. I really couldn't numb myself and so instead I had to feel everything, and that taught me the meaning and real example of letting go.

Sometimes I feel pain so deeply and so hard it seems like I weep for humanity and for eternity. But if I don't do that, the pain actually hurts me now. I put this down to how long I withheld things in previous years and just didn't know how to express myself, nor did I feel safe to do so.

At first, I was cleaning up my life for someone else—my unborn child. I started with what I thought was my first, biggest, and final clean up. Then I would get pregnant. For me that was smoking—smoking to bring peace. I tried several times and realized just what a hold it had over me. I sought help and I did it. Next, it was stuff like my diet and paying more attention to my body and learning more about my monthly cycles. Once I had set this clear intention of cleaning up, the right people, the right books, the right webinars came in. It was all so new for me and I really did enjoy the lessons as I could apply them and they made sense.

I was doing my job at the time purely for the maternity rights. As I started to loosen my grip on having to stay just for the medical benefits, I decided to change my job. When I reflect back now, I can only smile at what the Universe had in store for me. Not because it was my "perfect" job, but because it opened doors for me and I met new people including Rachel.

Did I skip through my fertility journey, take it all in my stride? NO. Add into this a sense of control and entitlement. "I am doing all this and therefore I should get what I want when I want it and I am ready now." The disappointment of not conceiving brought some deep dark beliefs to the surface. Without the support of the Heart Led Living (HLL) community and my coach, Sue Dumais, I really don't know where I'd be now. I essentially believed, "I am not okay. I don't deserve good things to happen. I am a victim of life. I am being punished for being myself."

The stages of cleaning up that I mentioned weren't neat in the sense of one month addressing the diet, the next sorting out the job, then my thoughts. It was all a process, all an experience, like a life classroom, and I was given the time I needed to practise and really learn the lessons and make the mistakes. At times, I felt hopeful and other times I despaired. When I'd find out I wasn't pregnant in the early days, there were times I'd go out and drink to punish myself and also as a way of temporarily numbing what was so painful. This was probably the first time in my life I was really feeling and I couldn't always handle it.

I was so angry with the Universe at times. "All I want is this. What more can I do? I don't want material stuff like XYZ. I'm not hurting anyone." Stomp, stomp, and so on. I thought a child would give me purpose. I had to start loving myself, loving my body, and looking at the darkness that consumed me each month when I realized I wasn't pregnant.

I learned how not to live for the end of my menstrual cycle—the optimal pregnancy testing date. I learned I couldn't control my body. And I was also shown all the other areas of my life where I was thinking I was in control. At first, this was an incredibly painful revelation. There wasn't much I thought I couldn't control. I had to learn differently. Enter the people in my life to teach me the tools to unlearn everything I thought I knew.

The Confusion and the Clarity

The confusion can be summarized as "How am I going to get pregnant? How am I going to do this authentically and truthfully?" Using some of HLL's intuitive heart tools, I knew I was going to get pregnant, I knew Brett was the dad, and I knew I was gay and in love with a woman. My mind just couldn't figure this out, even though my heart could. What a control conundrum. So the confusion in my head was massive and this is an understatement. Add into this the time pressure I was aware of with my own body clock.

Dropping into my heart space, however, I just knew these three things. At one point in my life, I really couldn't get my head around (the irony!) that dropping into the heart is not actually New Age woo woo. It's actually our own internal GPS and, therefore, the only truly sane way to live our lives. So my head was full of confusion, and my heart was full of clarity.

I was so clear what I wasn't going to do: I wasn't going to lie to anyone including myself. I was also so clear of how I wanted to be: truthful and respectful. I was also certain that in my heart nothing was wrong, yet obviously my head was seeing only the opposite.

The connection with Rachel was whole.

My current relationship just wasn't right anymore. And I could not nor did I wish to devalue the fourteen years Brett and I had been together.

I was clear—this wasn't going to be an affair. I was now in a place in my life that I knew where to go for support and where not to go. There was no drama. I had no bad habits of numbing to fall back on. On reflection, the process was truthful, bold, and simple, and those involved could trust my honesty.

The feeling of Love won and was in my driver's seat. We really do have all the answers and knowing inside us and we only need to know the next step.

Clearing My Path

As I started shining a light on the areas of my life that needed clearing, I started to live more authentically and face the areas where I wasn't being authentic, where I was numbing my feelings. I was committed to doing this and I still am. In the early days of my fertility journey, I used to hope for an end to all my problems and challenges. I really do know that life just isn't that; life is an opportunity for growth. For me when I soften and surrender to what is, I feel safe and strong and I know what to do, what to say, and what not to do. I know where to reach out for the support I need and I know what the next step is on my path.

Sue Dumais and I had a conversation during my fertility journey. I was coming to terms with what was happening in my life. Sue had been in my life for a couple of years as my mentor and coach and someone I have the utmost trust in. She is the person I can go to, the person who helps me be responsible for my own stuff rather than projecting it all out there, which is so common in our culture. Sue has shown me how to face my fears, feel the feelings attached to them, and to release them so that I can return to and re-learn my natural state of inner joy and peace. As founder and leader of the HLL community, she holds us wholly accountable to healing our past wounds and our limiting beliefs, and to seeing things from a different perspective. She told me that my Spirit Baby was waiting and saying "Clear your path." I knew what that meant, as there was nothing else to clear.

My connection to the HLL community is solid. So I will clear my path. I was committed and in a place of blind faith—everything I had tried hadn't worked and everything I had tried to control was or had unravelled. I also wasn't being asked to do something "bad".

I wanted to live authentically and peacefully in every area of my life.

So allow me to walk you through that part of my life's path. These events all happened close together. I get goose bumps recalling them:

By this time I'd not given up on being pregnant. I think it was more like putting it on hold. Along with this, I was relaxing into what was happening and I was required to focus on each and every new step as it was all so new. I stopped counting the days, eating and living carefully yet rigidly. So I do recall drinking coffee, eating goat cheese, and painting my toenails as I reentered my life. I suppose in summary, my life had become broader than my fertility journey; however, that doesn't diminish the importance of becoming pregnant. I had to focus on my relationship with trust and faith, step by step. I had to honour my truth, not knowing the outcome, taking a step away from just being pregnant.

Rachel and I arranged to meet to talk. Both nervous, both excited, both honest, and vulnerable at the enormity and simplicity of what was. We walked and talked, something I find so therapeutic and expansive and something I apply in my coaching business with my clients when possible. Canadian author Danielle LaPorte talks about "core desired feelings" and I really relate to this as a way for a person to review and live each area of their life.

We talked about our feelings—my core desired feelings were Brave, Feminine, Love, Vibrant, and Abundance. What I knew for sure was I felt all five and could define each one. We didn't make plans; we "just" talked about how we felt. We kissed.

I am so proud of myself for how I chose to tell Brett. I knew I needed to, I wanted to, I was scared to, and I could acknowledge that I didn't want to "lose" him. He was so important in my life. He is such a great guy, but I knew I had to tell him. I knew I was, in one sense, freeing us and, in another, severing something. Clearing my path in this moment meant clearing my fears and my attachments so that I could do the right thing. I did not know how he was going to react. He had been my rock for so long. Where would I be without him?

"I love you, but I am not in love with you. I've fallen in love with a woman."

To this day, I am in awe of and humbled by his dignity, his response, his actions, his self-respect, and self-love. He emanates a kindness and an acceptance of life. If it had been the other way around, I cannot guarantee or envisage I would have delivered a consistently mature or dignified response. My respect for Brett in how he heard and honoured himself in that conversation will always stay with me. We were in new uncharted territory. I was in open communication with Rachel and Brett about the way forward.

Not long after telling Brett, I did a pregnancy test, as my period was late, very late actually. This was the first month in a long while I'd not noticed or charted which day I was on. There was no reason to check. I couldn't fully see the stick to double check it as my eyes were brimming with tears. It was positive. I was pregnant. I had been truthful, I was in love, Brett was the dad. I had cleared my path and I realized that, physiologically, I could only have conceived before all of these events.

Brett was overjoyed—I could see it in every cell of his being. Not a sense of us getting back together; just a joy to learn he was going to be a dad.

I also enjoyed the joy that came. I had a deep respect for myself and the two people in my life. It was all about honour, trust, and transition.

I had to grow through a whole load of guilt and shame. I had to shed layers of the stuff and that was a process. That felt pretty scary and debilitating, and for me that is where my HLL coach and the HLL community come in as a neutral, safe space to just be, to be challenged and heard without judgment and criticism.

Transitioning from Partner to Friend

Brett and I had been partners living together for almost fourteen years. We had just bought a house to be our family home. We tried to sell it not long after our conversation. It was a lovely house but the Universe had other plans. We then had another conversation about staying in it together as friends for the first year of Willow's life. Some of our friends had shared with us that the first year of a baby's life isn't easy and we would need one another's support. Also, there would have been a hefty financial penalty if we had cancelled our fixed mortgage agreement with just over a year remaining. Staying together came about as our house just wouldn't sell.

It's interesting—I remember thinking on our first date fourteen years before, "You will be a great dad." For sure, babies, settling down, and all that jazz were not on my radar then, but it's interesting that I thought that so clearly, particularly reflecting how my life has played out.

My pregnancy was calm, there were no complications with Brett, and I knew it wasn't going to happen again so I appreciated it, enjoyed it, and was really present to it all. I recall the yoga sessions and how sacred they were to me. I had already learned the effects of fear on my body and hers (all learned on the fertility journey). It really was a time to honour myself and her.

It was a private time. We don't live our lives on social media anyway but it really was a time when those involved grew and transitioned, and I played my part in this. There was no lying. I enjoyed being myself. It was a process and I chose to trust as the worry would affect both me and my baby. Trusting was non-negotiable.

The appointments were with Brett, we made decisions

together, and we were transitioning into a friendship. It was peaceful and honest and I felt safe. We had time to discuss the practicalities of equal parenting rights and responsibilities and helping each other out—great foundations that we live and breathe now.

I had to learn to make peace with not being in control, as you can see the plans had changed because I was listening. This was not how it was originally meant to be. This was, however, an exhilarating, peaceful, and loving time of my life.

Brett was at the birth of our daughter Willow Grace. My waters broke at Rachel's house during the night and Brett came to collect me—it was the first time they had met.

It gives me shudders to think if I had done this any other way. If I had tried to control any of this. Firstly, Willow might not have come. And secondly, I had experienced living with fear and, as I headed toward my fifth decade of life, I was tired of that.

Transitioning from Friendship to Marriage

My nine months of pregnancy were also my first nine months with Rachel and these were joyous, raw, vulnerable, times. We had a surge of new energy as soul mates. I realized I was completely in love with her and my body responded well to this. As we blossomed in private it allowed the fears of judgment to wash up. I allowed this each and every time. The more vulnerable we were with one another, the more our relationship and connection deepened.

Rachel had always lived independently and had chosen to be a solo mum with her own independent fertility journey. She lived with her young twin daughters. I was the first partner she had lived with. I'd not lived independently and I'd not lived with children before. I'd lived with Paddy my dog for ten years and this was the first pet Rachel's girls had lived with.

The first year of Willow's life, Rachel and I got to know one another and carved out regular time for one another. It was during this time we discussed joining our two units. Willow, Paddy, and me and Rachel, Niamh, and Elsa. In some aspects, it was a gentle and gradual process and we took the decisions affecting our nurturing responsibilities seriously. Knowing that I had the strength to open new conversations, own how I felt, and be brave in asking for what I needed, Rachel and I broached the subject of joining our lives at first hypothetically. "Can you imagine us ever living together? Can you imagine ever telling so and so that we are together?" It was a fun way to consider new ways of being.

Following the first year of Willow's life, Rachel decided to move into the home I lived in and Brett decided to move into the one Rachel lived in. Both houses had been on the market. They made these decisions independently. There was no rushing, no fear-based decisions; opportunities arose in a quiet calm flow. I was in awe during this time of what was happening.

Initially, it was just the two of us getting to know one another and falling deeper in love. So moving everyone in together was an adjustment in every respect, sharing a space together, making it a home for all six of us. It was also a time I had to let go of Willow, as she now had two homes. While Brett and I had discussed it so carefully, we knew we would see her very regularly, during "the other's week," it was still an emotional wrench initially. It's not that I didn't trust Brett—I attacked myself emotionally. "Am I a terrible mum? I am a part-time mum. This isn't how it should be. Willow is going to hate me." Others judged me too, how I should have stayed with

Brett purely for the sake of my child. I knew from experience that this was not true, but it hurt to be judged over something so emotional. I knew I had made the right decisions, but it was a process to grow through to fully believe without any doubt and grief so that I didn't project any of this on Willow or anyone else. I found the strength to accept that others would judge and criticize and see only drama. I am truly grateful to them actually for helping me see I was doing the right thing and learning from it. Other people's words could only trigger me if I believed them to be true.

It's fair to say I had to recognize and let go of my expectations and face my fears. Life is harder when you feel sleep-deprived, when a child is sick, when people feel disconnected because they are navigating life in their own, different ways. We were learning to share a space, to lean on one another, to ask for support, and to redefine what family and home mean to us.

Rachel and I have transitioned into blending our two families into one unit and one union: Rachel, her twin daughters Niamh and Elsa, me, my daughter Willow (our dog Paddy has since passed on). Our daughters' acceptance from the beginning just gave greater weight to our certainty. We could have had resistance and drama and we didn't. Yes, we had new considerations, with two strongly independent women running a home together.

We chose to get married in 2017 as we headed toward our three-year anniversary. We chose to do it our way, no frills, no fuss, just "I do" at an intimate ceremony with a few friends as witnesses. Our wedding vows were a commitment to friendship, love, and support. Everything stems from these values.

We used the same kind of process we'd used in clearing our own paths—answering why we are doing it, what fears we have, others' expectations, what feels right, and what brings us joy. Yes, some people are disappointed with how my life is—I've been told I must be feeling bereft! I'm learning to make peace with that. Our children have just gone with the flow and accepted what is—they have two mums who are in love, doing their best to demonstrate what love is, and they live in a place of honesty, safety, and joy. Willow has two homes like this and an amazing dad. Remember, there is no rule book! The boundaries blur over time, the black and white areas soften into grey as we nurture ourselves, our children, and our home. Sharing decisions, insecurities, perceived weaknesses, deepening into what it really means to be patient, compassionate, loving, honest, letting go, and trusting.

The Closet

It's not until I realized I had been living in a closet that life became scary. Once I became aware I had been, it was as though a light was being shone on me and I had a choice of what to do. A metaphor could be that of a butterfly coming out of a cocoon. I am so grateful to have a core group of dear friends and my dear brother with whom I could actually share my whole story—to practise speaking my truth. The story I am sharing with you here. I wept as I said, "I am pregnant. I've split up with Brett but we are cool and we are friends and soon to be parents. And I am in love with a woman. Her name is Rachel and she is a solo mum with twin girls. So, yes, I am gay."

I remember now it was as if my life was triangular. For my trusted circle and HLL community it was only complete to share the three aspects. And the weeping was so cathartic with each friend. It was joy, awe, relief, and gratitude.

For most, though, it was just the first part of the news—the story of pregnancy only and that is fine too. While I cannot control how others hear or respond in a way that I want them to, it was a great time for me to practise discernment about what I shared.

During my maternity leave I felt so protected, in an expansive cocoon. Tending to these new relationships was sacred and important, as well as tending my relationship with myself from maiden to mother. We did things our way and in private. My roles were evolving at the same time and I enjoyed them. Co-parent, mum, partner. Everything was new, there was no rule book other than the values of trusting and feeling and listening. I had the space and time to have lots of sweaty-palm conversations and process my feelings around them in order to continue clearing my path.

As the time came to return to the job that was paying my maternity leave, I realized just how my life had and was continuing to transform. The house exchange was arranged. Rachel and I worked together, so we knew a lot of the same people. I chose to tell some people directly—"There is something I'd like to share with you." With others I smoothly just dropped it into conversation. I was using the word "girlfriend." Other times I felt floored by the fear of gossip and judgment. I grew stronger and more confident over time and really was proud of who I was and who I was with.

Rachel and I would laugh. "Who have you told today? How?" It's not like I turned into an extrovert and started posting my life on social media, but she knew it was part of my process. I was experiencing how to live unapologetically and follow my intuition as to what to say, not say, when, and to whom.

Not long afterward, I left this job as I was meant to return to my coaching business, which I'd reduced during maternity leave. The job and the people had, as with everything, given me the opportunity to grow, shed, be authentic, and enjoy being and becoming myself.

It's necessary to come out because it's okay. It's okay for me to blossom into who I am. I cannot and will not apologize for who I am, only for things I have done, and I am willing to course correct as I go.

The Experience Matters

With a clear creative mind you get clear directions.

The more whole I am the more fulfilled I am. I am not broken and don't believe anyone else is either; nor do I need fixing. The hope that I could be any different is just insanity. I found the missing piece; I found peace. I wasn't losing something; I was gaining something—my choice, my curiosity, my discovery, my expression of who I am, and who I am becoming, becoming whole. Remove the definitions for who you are and see where that takes you.

There is no rule book. Be at the helm of your life. Live your expectations, boundaries, and freedom.

I return to the tree where I received Rachel's first email alone and with my family. I see it in all its seasons. I have a badge that says "Imagine Peace." I've crossed out "imagine" and written "choose" on the badge. I choose peace. My title of "Black and White to Rainbow" really reflects me seeing how I was so rigid and with that came only judgment and criticism. "This is how it is; it isn't; it should be; it shouldn't be." I'm learning to change how I perceive the outside world and paying close attention to monitoring my inner world.

How different this could all have been. Removing my definitions has allowed me to navigate what could have been a soap opera fraught with drama and pain. I shifted out of black and white and I'm okay with feeling. How do I want to feel and what do I mean by that word in each context? What do "love" and "brave" mean in this situation?

What if I am loveable? What if nothing is wrong? What if I'm not right? What if I can release my agenda and trust in something much bigger than I can imagine? What if I can choose peace rather than just imagine it? What if I am enough just as I am? What if everything is as it's meant to be right now because otherwise it wouldn't be happening? What if I get to choose my response in every moment?

What if I am not my incessant thought chatter and inner critic? What if I can just observe and release these thoughts? What if I can drop my armour of defence and attack, and communicate from a place of neutrality?

What I've shared here are my life lessons. I'm still learning to apply them to my path and my perceived challenges now.

I think I was given such a stark cluster of miracles to make sure I really did get that I am worthy of them. I can fall back on them in times of being lost in the fog. I really can see how rigid and controlling I can be—perhaps not to anyone else but more in my thoughts and inner dialogue. I used to feel so weak, so helpless, so much of a victim that either numbing or anger gave me the illusion of peace or power. Life isn't fair or unfair; it just is and it will unfold. It's for me to take responsibility for myself, my thoughts, and my actions.

I don't always remember and I often sit and allow my darkness and fear to consume me and I'm learning I can even find peace and acceptance with that now! The thing is fear hurts now, so I don't usually camp out in it so long. I am truly grateful that this chapter of my life is teaching me these lessons of how I want to be and equally how I don't, so I can apply them and teach them to others.

I invite you to consider my questions for your life right now. I clear my path with the freedom they bring me through each life challenge; I will continue to do so. What a humbling message and gift from my child Willow.

Some people have said, "Wow, you could make a film!" My response is that it is an incredibly powerful journey and story, but it is not a drama and that's a choice. Love is limitless. It's just an expression of who we all are. Natural. Simple. This is for sure the most peaceful chapter of my life so far.

My Reflections

There was a point in this story where I actually had to say to Sue, "I need to stop saying 'I can't believe this is happening.'" She gave me the reframe: "Say, 'I am in Awe'" Yes, that is it. I am in Awe.

If this part of my life's story had a voice, these are its messages and lessons.

It could have turned out so differently if I'd been afraid of my own shadow. It's okay to be yourself; be authentic, be who you are, don't give away your power. People-pleasing is just ugh. Acceptance of what is and who I am and therefore who everyone is. I'm okay and not broken.

Love in thought; love in action. Love is not just a noun; it's a verb. I cannot possibly be a loving presence in the world, if my internal world has self-hating thoughts.

Feelings are meant to be felt, honoured, and cleared, not numbed so they don't go anywhere. Once I feel behind the words, they no longer grip me. I had to stop numbing. I had to start feeling. Feelings were too painful for so long. I'm learning to shed what was running the show. Life gives me challenges. I can control nothing and no one, and I get to choose whether I want to live from a place of receptivity, trust, and love or from fear, pain, control, and punishment.

I don't need anyone's approval or disapproval. This is a great lesson for me to learn as a parent and for how I help nurture those around me to listen to and trust their own inner guidance. I accept I am not responsible for someone else's pain and choices, and they are not responsible for mine.

Closing my heart hurts now. I seem to have chosen a life in two halves. The first I numbed. I believed it truly was a harsh universe out to punish me. I live in the two contrasts. I can have hard conversations. I can allow myself space and do the same for others. I can clear my path to know and listen to what I am to do. I have found my people, my support, my sacred space—people I can trust in and who teach me to trust and listen to my intuition.

I'm getting to know my inner world. Get to know yourself. This is ongoing.

Was it easy to accept myself? How have I moved from an absolute NO to now?

For me, I journal it out, and then burn it.

I have core people to whom I can express where I am at.

I don't want this story to read like a happily-ever-after, as for me it's more about being comfortable to be and surrender to what is. I am willing to expose the Truth, to ask for support, to unwind from what was to what is, to really question how parenting should be done, and to ask what a family should look like. I'm willing to look at, expose, and own my fears, as I know they only weaken me otherwise. I am one of three adults who played their part in navigating these changes peacefully, maturely, carefully, and considerately.

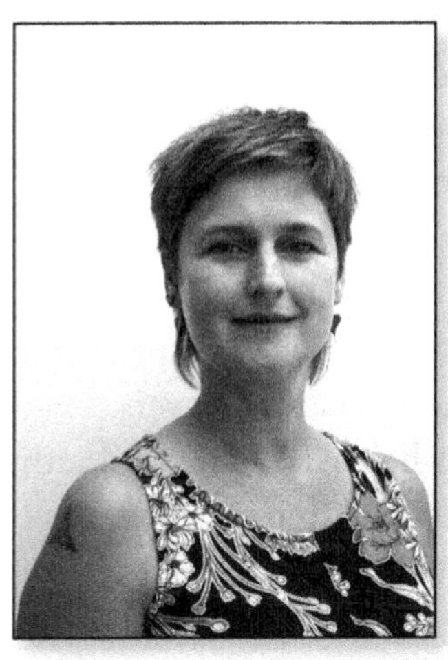

Author Biography for Kirsty Peckham, Intuitive Coach and Personal Transformation Coach

Kirsty Peckham is a Certified Intuitive Coach trained through Heart Led Living who works locally and internationally with women to help them find their inner peace and regain their balance.

Born in England, Kirsty has always been drawn to study and work in roles that enhance someone's life and community. She focuses on bringing positive development to the people and world around her. Her focus was originally on the world "out there." In travelling to various places in the world, she always had the deep desire to find peace and somewhere to belong. When she decided to really review her own life in 2012, she began to realize and face some of her inner turmoil and darkness that were consuming her life's choices, actions, and beliefs. She is part of this collaborative book to share her story of contrast from facing and stepping through the inner darkness to supporting herself and others who are ready to move through the crippling, inner turmoil, and step into their greatness.

As an intuitive coach, Kirsty focuses only on the now, not on rules or goals and, therefore, not on restrictions. She shows her clients how to tune in and trust their own intuition. She has a natural ability to create a sacred space where they feel safe and heard. She uses her intuition to guide them through the blocks they are not seeing.

She teaches others how to be captivated by true Love so

that their heart flutters and they feel alive inside. She is straight talking and works with people who are ready to release the stuff that is no longer serving them and who are ready to experience the inner peace that is our birthright. She creates a genuinely collaborative relationship with her clients as she knows all the answers are inside them; they just need the safe space and neutrality to locate and connect to their personal power.

The Heart Led Living community helps her seek her Truth and challenge her agenda—the bits she knows about and resists, and the deeper bits that she often doesn't even realize are running her life choices.

This community challenges her to take the next leap of faith, to grow, to expand, and to see things from a different perspective, so she clears her path and can be of service in helping others do the same to discover and rediscover their gifts. Kirsty lives in Eastbourne on the South Coast of England with her wife Rachel and their three children.

To learn more about Kirsty and her offerings, visit thecoachbythesea.co.uk.

Chapter 9

Welcome Me

by Joanne Sissons

Welcome Me

by Joanne Sissons

I Want to Be a Mother

I want a baby. I want to be a mum. I want to be like all my friends. They can have children. Why can't I?

These looping thoughts were all that I heard inside my head for almost four years. They were my first and last thoughts every day and I knew that I wasn't alone. I could see others seeking a child—the desperation was etched all over their faces. But it was crippling me. It had me spiralling out of control and lost in the darkness. At my lowest point, I imagined myself jumping off London Bridge into the Thames. That's what infertility did to me. It made me feel worthless as a woman, as a wife.

I'd spent thirty years perfectly happy without children, but as soon as I got married it became all that I could focus on.

I certainly didn't expect to get pregnant straight away, but I didn't expect the rollercoaster, soul-searching ride that I was about to embark on.

I've always wanted to be a mother. Some people aren't programmed that way, but I knew from an early age that I really wanted to have a family. When things were taking slightly longer than I had hoped and all my friends were becoming pregnant, I started to pay attention to my monthly cycle. It wasn't monthly at all. Sometimes, it was absent up to sixty days. Excitedly, I would pee on sticks in the hope that I was pregnant, but it slowly began to dawn on me that I needed to investigate what was going on.

Down to the doctors I trotted and that was when all the fertility prodding and devastating results began to consume my consciousness. Irregular periods, a low egg count for my age, and the signs of an early menopause gave me just a 5 percent chance of conceiving. I had become a number, an extremely low statistic that had been stamped on my brain forever. It still rings in my ears, way more than the word "menopause."

Trying In Vitro Fertilization

Disregarding this figure, we agreed to try a round of in vitro fertilization (IVF); it was way too soon to give up. I had a love-hate relationship with the amount of fertility drugs I had to take and was never at ease swallowing them. At my initial egg count scan, when my egg count should have increased because of the fertility drugs, I remember waiting nervously with my mum to be called. We stared at the screen while they performed the scan, only to be faced with an image of two empty ovaries. Yep, nothing. Not even one little egg. The nurse looked concerned. My mum wanted to bundle me up and protect me. And I fell, like a crumpled mess, to the floor. My husband rushed home from work and I broke down in his arms.

This was the first time I mentioned to my husband a vision I had had of a little boy. "But, honey, I think we are meant to have a boy," I sobbed.

This sentence was met with silence. My husband never once encouraged me to believe this. He saw my pain and didn't like me to hold onto something I may or may not have seen. That was his role throughout our fertility journey. He always supported me emotionally and never put pressure on me to have a family; I did that to myself. He was my rock and I'll be forever grateful for this.

Despite my empty ovaries, my obsession with wanting a baby grew more intense. I tried almost every fertility therapy in the hope of improving my eggs: acupuncture, reflexology, plenty of herbs, even a holiday. Whoever says "go away and relax" to a woman trying to conceive should think again. It doesn't matter where you go in the world, your thoughts go with you. There's no place to hide. I threw thousands of British pounds sterling at my desperation. I even tried another round of IVF at one of the top London fertility clinics.

"If That's What You Want to Do"

The doctors finally advised us that egg donation would be my best chance. I'm one of three girls, so my initial thoughts were, "Phew, perhaps they can help." But to my utter surprise it was my best friend and creative work partner who offered. It was perfect. We look similar, we have the same beliefs, and my mum calls us "soul sisters." It was the most beautiful gift a friend could ever offer.

I remember cautiously telling everyone who mattered to me about the idea. My husband was open, my mum was delighted, my sisters said, "It makes sense; she looks more like you, than we do." But it was my dad's words that didn't sit well with me.

Dad was diagnosed with multiple sclerosis (MS) when I was fifteen. We witnessed him being whipped in and out of hospital, and his body slowly being taken away from him. He was an incredibly proud Welshman who refused to be beaten by the disease. Every time he was admitted into hospital, instead of taking the easy path and not returning to work, he went back to work. His fight with his illness was both courageous and determined. But when he did finally retire, and my mum was struggling to look after him at home, he gave in to the idea of going into a care home. Guilt ran through my mum, but ultimately they both knew it was for the best.

Every time I visited him there, I saw him slowly surrendering to the disease and his destiny. He had found a peace that I had not seen in him before. He was a man of very few words, but his speech was disappearing, he had little movement, and in the end he was fed through a tube. One day when mum and I had done our general fussing over him, silence fell in his room. I filled the void with my news of implanting my friend's eggs, assuming he would just nod his head with approval, but to my surprise he managed a full sentence. "Well, if that's what *you* want to do."

I wanted to scream. I didn't know if that's what I really wanted. I just felt utter despair and I didn't know how else I was going to achieve a family. But that was it; end of conversation.

We carried on with the egg donation regardless, until one evening I heard Sue Dumais on a fertility web seminar saying, "Listen to your heart. What does it want you to do?"

I was instantly gripped. I knew I had to stop everything—all the fertility appointments. And the kindest gift that anyone could ever offer me. I simply couldn't make my best friend go ahead if I wasn't one-hundred percent sure. I had to find out what my heart had been whispering while my head had been shouting.

Everyone who had supported me on my desperate quest to have a baby was surprised and a bit disappointed when they found out that I'd said no to my best friend. My husband questioned whether I was sure; he just wanted me to be happy. My mum was upset; she was so keen for me to experience life as a mother, just as she had. These reactions made me question my decision, but no, I felt at peace, and that's when I knew deep down in my heart that I had made the right decision. Now, I needed to delve further into what was blocking me from successfully having a baby.

I Was Still "Wanting"

I reached out to Sue and with her help I made some life-changing discoveries. I say life-changing, because I am still very passionate about this subject and I would like to assist others on their fertility journey.

I began by looking underneath each of my "wants." Instantly, it became crystal clear that they were blocking me from creating a new life. Each want was filled with fear and worry.

1. "I want a baby." But I didn't believe I could get pregnant because I had hooked onto all the horrifying medical results.
2. "I want a baby." But I had a deeply rooted fear that my baby was going to have MS.

This was big. My constant wanting had all been in vain,

utterly pointless. The truth was I was terrified and full of self-doubt. My thoughts had blocked any connection to my womb, leaving it feeling cold and unloved from all the devastating medical results. But it was the gateway to having a baby. I needed to love it, not hate it. Sue encouraged me to visualize my baby and welcome its soul into my womb. This took time. I found a fertility massage clinic to help me look inward and reignite my womb.

The fear connected with my second "want" was an energy cord that ran deep between me and my dad. MS is not considered hereditary, so why was I thinking it was? Underneath this layer was the belief that if I had a child, this crippling disease would take away someone else that I love. This energy cord that I had unintentionally created over time between me and my dad needed to be cut. So with Sue's help I freed myself from this belief. As I visualised myself cutting the cord, suddenly, my whole body shook from head to toe. An intense amount of energy was rising up and out. I felt embarrassed that I couldn't control my shaking, but Sue reassured me that the energy needed to be released and to let it flow. When I did eventually come to stillness, I felt a freedom that I hadn't felt for a long time. I had released the connection.

My infertility was shedding light on areas of my life that I needed to expose and heal. Breathing into and witnessing these blocks, I was beginning to feel a shift. Now, I was ready to see what my heart was saying.

Visions of a Spirit Baby

Images of our baby boy appeared sporadically at first and I quickly dismissed them. Nobody told me to hold onto them or to believe in them until I met Sue. Together we tuned into the energy that surrounded my body. There, sitting in a green ball of pulsing light on my right shoulder, was my baby boy. Tears streaked down my cheeks as I felt into the gentle pulse that connected us. "Is he a boy?" I tentatively asked, thinking she might think I was crazy for sharing this vision.

"Yes" said Sue.

My heart melted. My visions were messages from my heart. There was a boy for us; I just had to believe.

Sue explained that the visions I had been experiencing were of my baby in spiritual form. She explained that such a baby is known as a spirit baby who has consciously chosen its parents. A spirit baby can hang around its mother and father for months or even years before choosing to leave the comfort of its spiritual world. Such babies are keen communicators as long as we are open to receiving their messages. Communication can come through images, signs, colours, and certain words that will stand out while we're reading. These messages can be subtle, but they are reassuring signs that your little one is with you.

Communication started flooding in once I had decided to step into the belief that my spirit baby was with me. One night I felt his legs wrap around my hips. Another time he popped up in between my husband and father in-law at a restaurant. I felt his presence in the new house that we had bought in Kent, and my pulse quickened with his excited energy when we were at the local nature reserve. I was receiving more and more detail; I was getting to know him. Blue eyes, blond hair, and he liked fishing just like his dad. I often found myself drawing sketches of him. I enjoyed his presence; it was a reminder to stay inward and positive.

"We Welcome You"

Slowly I was beginning to feel a softening around my fertility journey. I was consciously surrendering to everything that had happened and anything that might yet happen. I was beginning to feel unattached to an outcome and, with that, I felt a sense of peace within. Every time I picked up that the "wanting" had returned (and I did), I knew I had shifted out of my heart and into my head, into my egoic mind. The ego mind thrives on fear and judgment and wants us to find answers quickly, but the heart has a deep sense of knowing. So, I began to swap the word "want" to "welcome." It may sound like such a simple idea, but at the time it brought about a huge shift; it was my saving grace.

Let's look at these words for a moment. When you hear the words "I want a baby," how do they sound to you? Putting my attachment to this sentence to one side, for me they sound sad, demanding, and full of desperation. Another meaning of "to want" is "to lack" or "to be without something desirable or essential." Every time I said, "I want a baby," all the Universe could hear is "I lack a baby. I lack what everyone else has. I lack fulfilment."

The ego mind wanted me to latch onto this lack and to listen. But these negative thoughts weren't serving me anymore. I consciously decided to switch them *off*.

Now, take a moment and feel into this sentence, "I welcome a baby." How does this sound to you? Can you discern the difference that it brings, not just to the mind, but to the physical body? Other meanings of the word "welcome" are "to greet, to invite," and "to allow." The Universe hears this sentence as a warm embrace and creates a softening in our heart, a welcome space in our body. Spirit babies want to know that they are welcome to join their prospective families; some need a compassionate hand to reassure them that they can make the leap when their time is right. Everyone loves to feel loved, even a spiritual one.

I found a mantra that I repeated every day to help me stay in this compassionate space. “We love you. We welcome you. We’re ready when you are.” This mantra was incredibly powerful for me. Whenever self-doubt reared its ugly head, I found myself coming back to my mantra.

This mantra had two parts. The first part was filled with love, a welcoming message. The second part—“We’re ready when you are”—was a reminder that we are not in charge of when a spirit baby chooses to arrive; they are.

I had been so wrapped up in time. My husband and I were getting older and I wanted a baby quickly before we got too old. But spirit babies don’t have the same concept of time that we do. They may have something to do before they arrive like transition with a family member. Everyone comes into this world with a predesigned plan and in divine timing. This part of the mantra helped me let go of time and give the control back to our spirit baby.

Our Spirit Baby Is Here

I’ll never forget the day I found out I was pregnant. It was the day after my best friend, the girl who had offered to be our egg donor, announced that she was pregnant with her second child. I was delighted for her, but I was kicking myself. Why hadn’t I proceeded with her offer? My opportunity had gone. I’d been such a fool to trust!

The next day, my husband and I were up at the crack of dawn to drive to Devon for a surfing trip. While he strapped the surfboards to the roof of the car, I nipped into the bathroom and, for some reason, I did a pregnancy test. I’d done hundreds before and I just expected the same result. But my heart raced when I checked. Our baby was here. It had decided *now* was its time.

My husband couldn't believe his eyes when I showed him and he made me do several tests to confirm the results. My mum broke down with joy and prayed, thanking the Lord for answering her prayers. Remaining proud, my dad tried to hold back the tears and my sisters were very surprised. My in-laws cried and did what they do best, popped open a bottle of bubbles. And my best friend jumped around and swore several times, way too many to count. We both laughed at how beautifully timed it was—we'd both be off on maternity leave from work together. It couldn't have been orchestrated more perfectly.

I kept up my mantra throughout my pregnancy; I was determined to stay connected. I loved my ever-expanding belly. Pregnancy was finally a reality. This was our miracle.

I went over my due date by almost two weeks. Remembering that our spirit baby's energy had quickened at the nature reserve, I decided to go for a brisk walk around the lakes. I thought it might help our baby make the transition. Sure enough, I went into labour that evening and the following day, our blue-eyed, blond-haired baby boy arrived. Yes, a boy! My heart visions had come true.

Divine Timing

"Is he your first?" people would ask me as we attended the morning playgroups.

"Yes," I said, being so grateful for one. But this question assumes a couple is going to have more. Were we going to have another baby? I had learned so much about spirit babies and how to connect with them that I began to tune inward to see what my heart was saying. One afternoon I was playing with my son on the bed. I picked him up and without thinking said, "Where's your baby sister?" Oh, this was a message from the heart; we were going to have another baby, a girl.

I returned to work with my best friend, but I struggled. My heart was still at home. The struggle became even harder after celebrating our son's first birthday. He became unwell with a virus and was covered in spots. We just assumed it was chicken pox and looked after him at home. But one of the spots on his foot kept swelling. It became so badly infected that he couldn't walk on it, which was awful for him as he'd just learned how. We were quickly admitted to hospital. He had cellulitis, a painful and serious bacterial skin infection. The infection spread to both feet and he was on intravenous antibiotics solidly for five days. It was a highly stressful time for everyone, and I put thoughts of having another baby to the back of my mind. Slowly, the swelling went down on both feet, and the doctors cheered when he began to take baby steps again.

The day we took our son home was such a relief. As we drove out of the hospital carpark, my husband said, "Right, let's not go back there again for a while." I nodded, but intuitively I felt like we would be going back. Indeed, that evening my dad took a turn for the worst and was admitted into the same hospital. We went back and, sadly for us, Dad died the following week. I'll be forever thankful to my dad for holding on until our son had been discharged. My loyalties would have been spilt.

Dad's death was full of sorrow, but his quality of life had deteriorated and I found myself inviting him to leave. Quietly, I repeated reassuring messages, "You're welcome to leave, Dad. Don't hold on anymore; we'll look after Mum."

I was so proud of him for battling the disease for so long, but I didn't want to see him struggle any longer. The very last time I visited him, I witnessed his spirit sitting above his body. I looked down at Dad breathing shallowly on the bed, but that wasn't the courageous, proud man that I knew and loved. The soul of that person was floating beside us. I never told anyone else what I saw. I couldn't quite believe I had seen his spirit so clearly. Occasionally, Mum stroked his forehead and called out his name in a desperate attempt to invite him back. I watched as his spirit briefly thought about it, but just couldn't commit.

I asked Dad to wait until I had left before he passed away. I didn't feel strong enough to see him draw his last breath and, as if he heard me, he waited until we had all gone before he died.

"Tomorrow always comes," my mum used to say to me when I was in my darkest place on my fertility journey. She used to say it as an offering of hope. She's right. Life goes on even without a loved one.

Several weeks after Dad's funeral when I had returned to work, I was sitting in meditation when I received a vision of my belly pregnant. Excitement ran through me—this was another heart vision of a spirit baby. Yes, I was now ready to start welcoming another child to our family. I reached out to Sue for some help to clear everything that had just happened with Dad's passing.

I spent most of the session weeping and saying my final goodbyes. Then together we tuned into my spirit baby. Intuitively I opened my heart chakra and welcomed our baby to us. I felt a flash of white light—her soul—enter through my heart and settle within me. She was here. Feeling a sense of excitement and urgency I booked a fertility massage appointment to help me connect with my womb. I knew I had neglected it because of everything that I had been through.

When conception started to take longer than I hoped, the "wanting" ego mind and thoughts of just a 5 percent chance started to creep back in again. But no, not this time. I was quick to spot them and refused to latch on. This spirit baby had a connection with my dad and his passing. It felt as though he needed to transition before I conceived. I knew she was with me; I just needed to trust that everything was playing out perfectly.

Trusting in Our Baby

To our delight, several months later I did become pregnant, and once again the news was beautifully timed. It brought a new sense of purpose and happiness to my mum. She was struggling to find her role in life after Dad's death, and was undergoing some major joint surgery. Our exciting news gave her something to aim toward, a new grandchild to meet, love, and nurture. Then a couple of months later, my younger sister also announced that she was expecting. This provided Mum with an extra boost of energy to get her through the next hip operation. It felt like our babies' arrivals were answering my promise to look after Mum.

This pregnancy was different; the spirit baby wasn't as keen to communicate as my son had been. I found myself judging the silence, but I kept up a trust mantra: "I trust in you." I did receive a couple of heart visions—autumnal leaves being kicked, a love of colour and, in Savasana, yoga's final resting pose, I felt her energy dance around my right hip to the relaxing music. I was drawn like a magnet to anything pink and often came back from the salon with pink nails. The difference I experienced with this pregnancy taught me that even in spiritual form spirit babies have their own personality.

The trust that I formed with my baby became so deep-rooted that, although my husband wasn't sure, I kept receiving glimpses of us having a home birth. Our son's delivery wasn't smooth; we'd needed a team of professionals in the end to help. So my husband was fearful of a home birth. But I trusted that our baby and I knew exactly what to do. So, on one wet wintry night in November, I gave birth to our baby at home, in front of the log fire. To a baby girl. Yes, a girl! It was the most beautiful and empowering experience, one that I will *never* forget.

I feel incredibly grateful for believing in myself, and I often have to pinch myself when I watch my two children together. My heart visualizations have come true: my blond-haired, blue-eyed boy already loves fishing at the age of three, and his mood transforms when we walk around the nature reserve. It's too early to tell at just ten months old if our daughter will love autumnal leaves, but she's a happy soul who's keen to be part of the family. She's a reminder that physical babies and spirit babies are made up of pure love. They see everything through the lens of love; there's no fear or judgment of anyone or anything; they lead with their heart and have a strong desire to be loved. We were all like her, once.

Intuitive Fertility Coach

I hope my story can bring some comfort to others struggling to conceive, or to others who may be yearning for something or someone new in their life.

For me, it was a baby, but now I find myself applying my six top tips that my fertility journey taught me to other aspects of my life. After sixteen years of working in media, I am starting something new, I am stepping into being an Intuitive Fertility Coach.

So, wherever you are on life's journey, here are my six top tips for you to reflect on:

1. Feel the power of welcoming.
2. Be willing to look underneath the fears.
3. Be open to your life lessons.
4. Trust that everything is playing out just perfectly.
5. Create a mantra.
6. Meditate.

Meditation can be a great way to go inwards. We spend so much time in our heads, looping 90 percent of the same thoughts as yesterday. Whether these are of a baby, a career or, of love, we become like stuck records. Meditation brings a stillness to the mind. It enables us to hear what the heart is saying.

For the last two years, I have been studying with Sue Dumais on the Heart Led Living Intuitive Coaching Program. Throughout the course, I have been receiving gentle heart nudges to be of service to others struggling to conceive, and these nudges have been getting louder. I can't ignore them any longer. The course has taught me to be a clear channel, to receive guidance from my heart, to share only what is guided, and to not give answers from the head, but to seek them from a place of knowing—the heart.

I didn't know that my life's path of desperation would bring me together with Sue, or that I'd be one of her Heart Led Living Coaches. But it's brought deep healing, miracles, and new intuitive gifts. Take a moment to reflect on your life's path. I wonder what your path is teaching you. You may not think so right now, but it's all purposeful. My journey certainly has been.

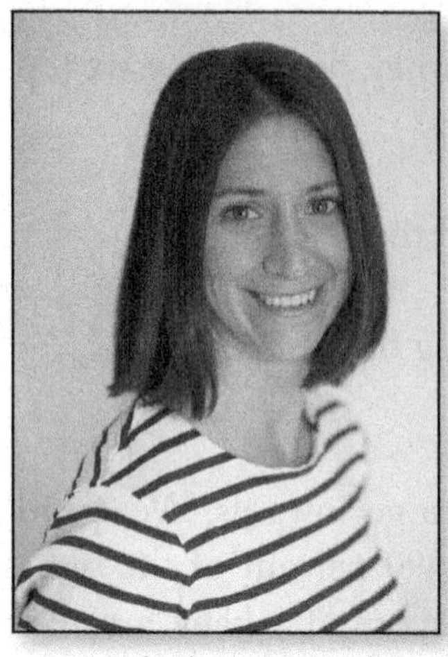

Author Biography for Joanne Sissons, Heart Led Living Coach and Intuitive Fertility Coach

Joanne Sissons lives in Kent, the South East corner of England. She's a multi-award winning creative working in London. But despite all her creative success, Joanne hit rock bottom when she and her husband received the news that she had just a 5 percent chance of conceiving a baby. Determined not to let her medical results be her destiny, Joanne looked for ways to improve her chances of having a baby. But it was only when she started to look inwards to her heart for answers that a shift started to happen. That's when her new passion for spirit babies and how to connect with them was ignited.

Joanne is a strong believer in mothers-to-be trusting their intuition, not their head or the medical profession. She believes that when we stop "wanting" and start "welcoming" our future baby to us, it can create a softness. A positive result. Working with her heart as her guide, Joanne began to go deep and connect with her spirit babies, she and her husband now have two very welcomed children.

Joanne would love to hear from you, if you'd like to shine a light on what could be blocking you from conceiving, and you are ready to start welcoming your future spirit baby to your family.

You can reach Joanne and learn more about her offerings at heartledliving.com/our-coaches/Joanne-Sissons/.

What NOW?

This is not the end of the story. This is just the beginning. Now it is your turn to integrate all the gems, insights, and aha miracles into your life so you can continue to experience and celebrate them.

Imagine your life as a classroom for your deepest healing and greatest awakening. As you bring the gifts you gained from reading this book into your life you make a conscious choice to heal, to feel, to awaken, to enliven your heart and soul.

Here are some questions to help you get the most of this book. They can also be used for other books, workshops and life experiences to find the deeper meaning and shift your perspective to one of gratitude and appreciation for all of life's events.

Heartwork: Inner Reflection and Integration

Start by reflecting on everything that stood out for you in reading this book. Take a deep breath and imagine bringing these things into your heart. Soften your mind and let go of the need to figure anything out in your head. Instead, imagine taking an elevator down out of your head and bringing your awareness into your heart. Take five deep breaths. Now, ask yourself these questions. Set the intention to allow the answers to come from your heart as they pop into your awareness. Go with the first answer that comes, even if it doesn't make sense.

- How do I feel in this moment?
- Is there something or someone in my life that is no longer serving my highest good?
- Am I willing to heal and release what is no longer serving me?

- What is the first step I need to take in order to release what is no longer serving me?
- What do I need to do, be, or have in order to support my healing so I will align with my deepest heart desires?
- Am I willing to play my part to fulfill my heart's purpose?
- What message does my heart have for me in this moment?
- In every moment ask your heart ... what now?

Our heart is constantly guiding, directing, leading us in every moment. It is up to us to get out of our head and listen to the whispers of our heart. Ask your heart, what now? Find stillness and listen with your inner ear. The answers we seek are all within our heart. Our heart knows what we need to do and when we need to do it. All the details will be given in the present moment. Everything we need to overcome any and all of life's challenges is available when we tune in and listen to our heart. The side effect of letting your heart lead you in every moment is miracles. The miracles are abundant and the more you celebrate them, the more of them you will experience.

To learn more about our Heart Led Living Community and Sue's offerings, visit heartledliving.com.

Photographer Credits

Kent Smith
Photo credit: Kevin Hill Photography

Delle Vaughan
Photo credit: Bob Carter

Diana Calvo
Photo credit: Leah Casto of Luxe Photography

Joanne Sissons
Photo credit: Michael Sissons

Kelly Van Unen
no credit author photo

Lisa Windsor
Photo credit: Rummy Evans of Bad Monkey Photography

Kirsty Peckham
Photo credit: Andy Morse

Kimberly Shuttleworth
Photo credit: Wendy Hord of Soul Photography

Sue Dumais
Photo credit: Adrienne Thiessen of Gemini Visuals Photography

Rachel Shoniker
Photo credit: Carla Elaine Photography

Lightning Source UK Ltd.
Milton Keynes UK
UKOW01f1408021117
312037UK00005B/52/P